How to Beat Arthritis
with Immune Power Boosters

How to Beat Arthritis with Immune Power Boosters

Carlson Wade

PARKER PUBLISHING COMPANY
West Nyack, New York 10995

Wade, Carlson
    How to beat arthritis with immune power boosters / Carlson Wade.
    p. cm.
    Bibliography: p.
    Includes index.
    ISBN 0-13-396458-2. -- ISBN 0-13-396441-8 (pbk.)
    1. Arthritis-- Diet therapy. 2. Arthritis--Alternative treatment.
3. Natural immunity. 4. Holistic medicine. I. Title.
RC933.W232 1989   89-8669
616.7'220654--dc20   CIP

ISBN 0-13-396458-2

ISBN 0-13-396441-8 PBK

PARKER PUBLISHING COMPANY
BUSINESS & PROFESSIONAL DIVISION
A division of Simon & Schuster
West Nyack, New York 10995

Printed in the United States of America

DEDICATION

To YOUR Health-Packed Years Ahead
with Freedom from Arthritis

ABOUT THE AUTHOR

CARLSON WADE is a leading medical-nutrition reporter, having written 24 books in the field of natural healing. His works are highly acclaimed and have been translated into French, Spanish, German, and Japanese. He is editor of the *Natural Health and Fitness Bulletin,* writes "Country Kitchen" for a leading health magazine, also a series of medical news columns for various periodicals. His writings have appeared in newspapers and magazines throughout the world. He makes frequent radio, television, and personal appearances. These efforts have earned him recognition as an accredited member of the American Medical Writers Association. Millions of readers have been helped by his nutritional discoveries as presented in his many writings.

Foreword

The greatest hope of any arthritis patient is to hear his doctor say, "You are in remission." Carlson Wade, in his practical and compassionate guide, shows how the arthritic can put this hope to work and achieve freedom from this formerly "hopeless" condition.

Although traditional arthritis therapies—medication, radiation, chemotherapy, and surgery—are frequently successful, they do not correct the cause of arthritis. This book taps into the newer scientific knowledge of the immune system, the body's own self-defense fortress against many illnesses such as arthritis.

This is only the beginning. Carlson Wade offers a dedicated approach to successful self-healing techniques. You'll learn how to use numerous adjunct therapies at your disposal to significantly increase your chances of beating arthritis with a boosting of your immune system.

Even such "wonder substances" as cortisone, interferon, and interleukin-2, thought to be available only through experimental programs, can be manufactured *by your body itself.* Carlson Wade shows how you can make use of certain foods, nutrients, physical therapy programs, and home remedies that will help regenerate a sluggish immune system. Almost immediately, your body's immune system creates an inner battle against the hurtful arthritis invaders. By strengthening your immune response, you bring about healing of this encroaching illness.

Your body has cured itself of many illnesses throughout your lifetime. You've just got to push the right buttons to do it again with arthritis.

Carlson Wade offers you the guidance and shows you the buttons needed to push for healing through the immune system.

Each chapter provides not only knowledge but also hope. Each case history illustrates that we all possess the substances, cells, and elements needed to bring on remission of arthritis.

The entire process is put in your hands, dependent only on your ability to push the right buttons by choosing the appropriate therapies and applying them with full dedication and conviction.

You can say "goodbye to arthritis" with the help of a powerful immune system. This book shows you how to do it. Why not take advantage of the substances your body and mind can create to beat arthritis with immune power boosters? You can make this good news happen!

H. W. HOLDERBY, M.D.

What This Book Will Do for You

One out of seven Americans suffers from some form of arthritis. The degree of severity varies greatly. For some people, it is just minor aches and pains. For others, some serious forms can be potentially crippling. Millions of dollars are spent each year to find the cause, treatment, and cures to relieve these painful ailments which affect some 37 million people. The numbers are growing. Are you now or will you become the next victim? How can you ease and erase your distress? How can you resist its threat to your health and lifestyle?

This overwhelming challenge is met with the discovery that you can beat arthritis with a boosting of your immune system. This fortress against disease is the key to prevention and ultimate healing of arthritis. With the use of nutritional therapies, improved daily living practices, the increase of some foods, and the avoidance of others, you can invigorate and strengthen your immune system to uproot and cast out all forms of painful arthritis.

Until now, the typical treatments for arthritis have been medication, surgery, radiation, and chemotherapy. Such traditional methods are often successful by themselves but they do not free your body from the grip of arthritis on a permanent basis. Drugs, for example, are so powerful, they may result in serious side effects, including damage to blood-forming tissues, lungs, liver, and kidneys. Each person's treatment program has to be designed on an individual basis. Since response to medication varies greatly, the risk of side effects is extremely high. Many an arthritis patient has pleaded, "Please tell me how to ease my pain without medications. Isn't there anything I can do to be free of this illness?"

This book was written to show arthritics of all ages that there *is* an alternative to dangerous chemotherapy. It concerns the cause of your arthritis—a weakened immune system. The book then explains in simple, step-by-step programs, how *you* can use the simplest of modalities to repair your immune system to ease pain and eliminate arthritis.

This book is unique from others in the same area because it shows how a rebuilt immune system is the solution to the problem of arthritis. The latest scientific research shows that the "missing link" in the jigsaw puzzle of arthritis is a defect in the immune system. Zeroing in on this target, this book describes program after program that helps supply this "missing link" to stimulate your inner defenses to overcome and remove arthritis invaders and help you enjoy freedom from this so-called "hopeless" condition.

In rheumatoid arthritis, for example, pain is only one symptom. There are many other reactions of this complex autoimmune disease. (An autoimmune disease is one in which the body's immune system inappropriately attacks the body's own cells. In rheumatoid arthritis, the joints and other connective tissues are the targets of the immune system attack.) Other symptoms include fatigue, weakness, and depression. Must you continue to suffer with this form or any other type of arthritis?

No, say many leading immunologists. This book is the first to describe how you can use certain foods to strengthen your immune system to ease the distress. Is arthritis an allergic reaction? The latest findings show that if you eliminate several foods, your immune system recovers and arthritis just goes away.

A vitamin found easily in everyday foods helps stimulate a sluggish immune system and creates corrective healing of this devastating illness.

This book is the first to show how you can use vitamins as pain erasers. Different dietary programs, beverages, elixirs of everyday foods (recipes given) stimulate the immune system to release certain hormones that actually erase pain—without any drugs!

Relief of pain and swelling can be accomplished when you use cell-cleansing programs, certain seafoods, and hydrotherapy as only some of the immune-reactivating methods to heal arthritis.

Did you know that you may have an "arthritis personality" ? With unique "stress busters" and "tension melters," and guidelines on having a smile on your face, you can "laugh away" your arthritis pain!

For many drug-taking arthritics, "pain killers can give you a pain!" Aspirin medications are more hurtful, in many cases, than helpful. This book shows how you can use non-drug home remedies to do the job of pain relief without any side effects. You can even rub away your pain!

A treasure of immune-alerting and arthritis-fighting programs are included such as postural advice, exercise, activity, and all-natural pain killers that use ingredients found in any pantry or that are available at your corner food market.

This book is the very first to link arthritis to a weakened immune system. It then shows you how to invigorate your body fortress so that you can free yourself from arthritis—for your lifetime.

Have you been told, "You'll have to live with your arthritis"? This book tells you, "With a powerful immune system available to everyone who follows these programs—you will be able to live *without* your arthritis!!" Turn the page and walk into a world that is free of arthritis . . .

Carlson Wade

Contents

4. The Miracle Vitamin That Lubricates Your Arthritic Joints 43

5. How to Use Vitamins as Pain Erasers 53

1

How Nutritional Immunity Heals Arthritic Pain

Martha J. was in distress as she sat opposite her doctor in the examining room. She looked perplexed as she asked, "You're taking me off the old drug and putting me on still another one?" The doctor gently reminded her, "The first drug wasn't helping." Martha J. agreed as she felt a painful spasm of her persistent arthritis and looked at her stiff fingers, unable to hold needle and thread without difficulty. "I wish we could find something to help heal the pain and take away my arthritis!"

After years of enduring arthritis stiffness and worsening pain, Martha J. decided to follow a new understanding of this condition that had helped tens of thousands of others be healed of arthritis; namely, correcting the nutritional deficiency that was responsible for a breakdown in her immune system. She tried a holistic or total body approach that would strengthen her immune powers, thereby uprooting and casting out arthritic symptoms. In a supervised 12-step program, she was soon able to move without spasms and enjoy flexibility of her limbs.

Within a few weeks on an immune-boosting nutritional healing program, Martha J. had conquered a condition that was formerly diagnosed as "hopelessly arthritic." Her immune system was strengthened and made resistant to the condition. Her natural resources helped her enjoy a pain-free lifestyle. Today she is totally free of all her arthritis symptoms!

1

A DOCTOR'S 12-STEP NUTRITIONAL IMMUNE ARTHRITIS DIET

Martha J. is one of thousands of arthritis-troubled patients who have been relieved of discomfort via stimulation of a sluggish immune system as part of overall treatment at a medically supervised clinic.

Patients with arthritis and neuromuscular diseases, or injuries or deformities of the spine or extremities, have been healed when immune therapy was used by Robert Bingham, M.D., at his Desert Arthritis Medical Clinic in Desert Hot Springs, California.

Dr. Bingham's 12-step diet is designed to alert the body's immune system and help the patient recover from arthritic distress. Here is the "preventive healing" diet that zeroes in on the immune system to create resistance and recovery from arthritis in a short time:

Step 1. Prepare and serve as many foods in their raw and natural states as possible. This includes fresh fish, vegetables, nuts, fresh whole milk, eggs, and natural cheese. Frozen fruits and vegetables are acceptable when fresh is not available. *Avoid* canned and processed foods, although canned tuna fish and salmon are acceptable.

Step 2. Every meal should have some protein-lean meat, cheese, fish, nuts, and beans. Drink two or three glasses of milk or buttermilk a day. The diet should include seafood and liver once a week and five eggs a week.

Note: When asked about the high cholesterol content of the meat and eggs, Dr. Bingham explained, "When it comes to diet, we like eggs because of their high protein content, their high natural hormone content, and their digestibility. If a patient is having high cholesterol problems, we would rather have him or her cut down on fats from salad dressings, fried foods, and bakery goods, and also reduce sugar and refined carbohydrate intake. We find that yucca extract (see below) also helps reduce cholesterol as does exercise, B-complex, and bran."

Cook protein foods at low temperatures since enzymes and trace mineral values are reduced when foods are heated above 120°F.

Step 3. Some fresh juice, raw fruits, or vegetables should be eaten at each meal. Wash produce thoroughly to eliminate insecticide residues. Peel apples, peaches, and pears.

Step 4. Avoid processed and hydrogenated or "hardened" oils and fats. Salad dressings should be made with natural vegetable oils, vinegar, lemon juice, yogurt, or homemade mayonnaise. Natural oils such as soya, safflower, peanut, and olive are acceptable in small amounts if you are not overweight. Vegetable oils are preferred for home cooking purposes. Avoid most margarines, some peanut butters, prepared pie crusts, restaurant-prepared French fries, and potato chips as they are prepared with hardened oils.

Step 5. Rancidity is particularly objectionable in foods used by arthritics. Vitamin E is rapidly destroyed by rancidity. Avoid bacon, sausage, commercial salad dressings, potato chips, and other such fatty substances since they cause rancidity in the system.

Step 6. Avoid foods and bakery goods that contain bleached white flour. Use unbleached whole wheat or other grain flours for cereals, breads, hotcakes, and the like. Wheat germ can be added in cooking as a natural source of B-complex vitamins, Vitamin E, and many minerals—2 to 4 tablespoons a day. TIP: One tablespoon of bran may be added to your diet daily. Home-mixed granola with bran is your best cold cereal.

Step 7. Avoid preservatives, artificial flavors, and colors in food products.

Step 8. Minimize refined carbohydrates, especially white sugar, candy, soft drinks, pastries, and desserts. Honey, maple, or raw sugar may be used with discretion.

Step 9. Coffee and tea are not recommended; if taken, do not sweeten. Cola drinks should be omitted because of their caffeine and chemical fluoride content. Alcoholic drinks are restricted because of the damage they do to tissues. Chocolate contains oxalates which interfere with calcium absorption and must be avoided.

Step 10. Avoid the "nightshade plants" (foods containing solanines and their products)—white potatoes, tomatoes, eggplant, and garden peppers. Included in the pepper family are the cherry, red cluster, bell, sweet, green, pimiento, chili, long, and red peppers. *Note:* Black or ground pepper, which comes from a tropical berry, is acceptable. Eliminate any processed foods containing potato starch or tomato flavoring.

Step 11. Tobacco in all forms carries toxic solanine and nicotine substances into the blood and tissues. These are especially damaging to muscles and nerve metabolism.

Step 12. Avoid contact with lead, especially auto exhaust fumes and gases from burning fuel. Wash hands after handling paints, insecticides, newspapers, and other printed materials.

Yucca Extract for Joint Stiffness

Dr. Bingham has found that this herb helps stimulate the immune response which is a key in controlling and healing arthritis. "Yucca extract helps prevent, reduce, or eliminate the pain, swelling, and joint stiffness suffered by arthritis victims. A controlled study reveals that it also can prevent and lower high blood pressure as well as high cholesterol and triglyceride levels in the blood."

The natural yucca extract comes from the yucca plant which flourishes in the southwestern deserts and Mexico. "Its therapeutic agent is a high concentration of steroid saponin, which acts in the intestinal tract to improve circulation and reduce abnormal fat content in the blood. It produces beneficial results for the arthritic joints with no harmful side effects."

How to Use: Dr. Bingham suggests every arthritic give it a trial as a means of stimulating the immune response. "Six tablets are recommended daily; take two tablets with each of your three meals. Improvement should be noted in three weeks and should reach its maximum level within four months. It may be taken in repeated courses to prevent a recurrence of symptoms.

Where to Obtain: In tablet form, without prescription, at most health food stores and nutrition centers.

Dr. Bingham has been able to restore flexibility, heal pain, and build nutritional immunity into his patients to resist arthritis with this 12-step program as part of a total healing treatment. Thousands have responded with a stronger immune system, the key to freedom from arthritis. The program is the basis of your personal goal to cast out this debilitating condition.[1]

THE "MISSING LINK" IN THE ARTHRITIS
JIGSAW PUZZLE

In order to recognize the role that nutrition plays in the effective healing of arthritis, it is helpful to understand the condition itself.

Molecular biologists have discovered that the body's immune system is involved in different types of arthritis. By nourishing the immune system, it is possible for the body's system to resist and reverse the progression of the insidious condition.

These nutritional programs and specific nutrients are called "biologic response modifiers." They are used to help provide a "missing link" in the arthritis jigsaw puzzle. A newer knowledge of the condition has found that a deficiency in the immune system has broken down defense barriers to admit illnesses and conditions such as arthritis. *In many situations, the use of a single nutrient has been able to correct the deficiency and promote healing of arthritis.* In other cases, an immune-boosting program is used to include a number of nutrients as well as foods along with holistic or total body techniques. The goal is to fit in the missing piece in the jigsaw puzzle and plug the gaps in the fortress against arthritis.

ARTHRITIS, PAIN, IMMUNE SYSTEM

"Why does it hurt?" is asked by every arthritic.

The answer is being heard more frequently. "A defect in the immune system."

---

[1] Robert Bingham, M.D., Desert Hot Springs, California. Personal communication.

Looking at Your Immune System

The defense (immune) system helps protect you from invasion by germs, bacteria, viruses, and other agents that could be harmful. The immune system consists of two components:

1. Alarm System. It identifies outside invaders in your body—similar to an alarm wired to the windows, door, and trunk of a car. This mechanism in your body is provided by white blood cells called "T" lymphocytes—*thinking* lymphocytes. In rheumatoid arthritis, these "thinking lymphocytes" mistakenly perceive that there is an enemy in your joint spaces and sound a "false alarm"—just as a car alarm will sometimes sound without apparent reason. The "false alarm" signals other white blood cells called "B" lymphocytes (*battle* lymphocytes) to go in and kill the perceived enemy in your joints.

2. Battle System. The "battle" lymphocytes fight back by recruiting mediators of inflammation—an interactive relay system of molecules, cells, and other substances designed to kill the enemy. The end result is a rush of inflammatory cells to the area where the false alarm has sounded. Inflammation produces the symptoms from which you seek relief—joint redness, swelling, warmth, pain, limitation of motion, and morning stiffness.

Your Body Attacks Itself!

Arthritis is identified as an autoimmune disease in which your immune system triggers an attack on body tissues. Your immune system responds directly against parts of your body itself.

The primary cause of arthritis is believed to be this breakdown in the body's defense system. How to repair the damage?

NUTRIENTS THAT BOOST IMMUNE STRENGTH

Nutrition is the key piece to the puzzle of how the arthritic process is triggered. A deficiency of one or more nutrients opens the way to an arthritis-producing reaction: the white blood cells, particularly T-lymphocytes, respond to a foreign substance (antigen) in and around the joints.

Byproducts of the immune reaction inflame the lining of the joint, the synovium, causing soreness and stiffness. The inflammation process also releases substances that gradually eat away at cartilage and joints.

Nutrients are needed to boost immune strength—to stimulate the sluggish immune system, to block the hurtful lymphocytes and strengthen the body's defense barrier against arthritic invasion.

THE VITAMIN THAT STRENGTHENS THE IMMUNE SYSTEM

Vitamin C is unique in being able to strengthen your immune system to resist and cast out the harmful invaders that are to blame for your arthritic distress.

Vitamin C enters into the bone marrow to initiate the formation of the T-lymphocyte cells which are then programmed to detect and destroy enemy substances. Vitamin C also mobilizes the B-lymphocyte cells to produce antibodies that neutralize and erase a wider range of pain-causing invaders.

This arthritis-fighting vitamin alerts the T-cells to activate the reproduction of B-cells residing in the lymph nodes which in turn manufacture antibodies or immunoglobulins. These are complex protein molecules designed to attack and destroy the pain-causing invaders. This nutritional fortification helps your immune system challenge and win the war against the arthritis invasion.

HOW A DAILY FRUIT DRINK HEALED "HOPELESS" ARTHRITIS

Morning stiffness kept Oscar A. in so much pain, he had difficulty in holding a spoon at breakfast. He faced job loss because his hands were unable to pick up tools or perform routine foreman functions at his northwestern lumber mill. He tried arthritis medication but effects were minimal and he developed headaches and digestive upset as a consequence. Oscar A. felt painful spasms when gripping the wheel of his car. Was he going to become an invalid?

The company sent him to a medical nutritionist who learned that Oscar A. had a deficiency of Vitamin C. The advice was to add 2 tablespoons (about 2,000 milligrams) of a Vitamin C powder to a fruit juice and drink daily. After seven days, he could awaken with joint flexibility so that he could hop out of bed, perform morning chores with pain-free hands and legs, and then drive to his job and work throughout the day—free from arthritis pain.

Oscar A. drinks his Vitamin C daily and jokes to his co-workers, "This is my arthritis medicine! It has no side effects either!"

How Vitamin C Drink Erases Arthritis Pain

The Vitamin C prompts the body to produce protective amounts of *interferon,* a pain-fighting and disease-erasing substance that alerts the T- and B-cells to cast out arthritic-causing enemies from the body. This tasty drink greatly enhances a process known as *phagocytosis* wherein the immune system sends in cells to the arthritic-infected areas to promote an efficient destruction of invading pathogens. Vitamin C then boosts antibody secretions which are used by your immune system to cool pain, restore flexibility, and knock out irritating substances that are causing abrasive arthritis.

The Vitamin C drink is unique because it speedily stimulates the production of the prostaglandin PGE1, a hormone-like substance that is needed to produce T-cells and thereby build up the body's natural defense mechanisms to resist and root out malignant cells.

Make Your Own Arthritis-Fighting Vitamin C Drink

The powder form of this immune-boosting vitamin appears to be more rapidly effective than tablets, hence its recommendation. It is available at almost any health store or large nutrition center. About 2,000 milligrams (read package label for potency) stirred into a glass of any fruit juice will help wake up your sluggish immune system and encourage an inner cleansing away of the harmful bacteria involved in arthritis pain. "A glass of Vitamin C a day will keep arthritis away" is often said by former patients.

MEDICINES AND IMMUNE SYSTEM

Medications have the ability to reduce, but not stop, the manufacture and threat of the mediators of inflammation working in your joint spaces.

Although medications may somewhat reduce the vigor and quantity of inflammatory cells released into the joint and provide some temporary relief, they do *not* cut off the stimulant for inflammation that determines how long the discomfort will last and how severe it will be. The reason is that the "false alarm" system remains unchanged.

The immune system is better bolstered with the use of nutritional and natural therapies that have the potential for turning off the "false alarm" system. These nutritional therapies help boost the immune system so it halts the progressive inflammatory course of the illness. When holistic nutritional therapies shut off this "false alarm," the inflammation disappears.

12 WAYS TO INVIGORATE YOUR IMMUNE SYSTEM TO FREE ARTHRITIC PAIN

Nutrition is one method of invigorating the immune system and casting out arthritic invaders. Because the immune system is a complex network of specialized organs and cells, it is helpful to use an assortment of modalities to enhance the healing process.

Here is a set of 12 steps that help strengthen your immune system to fight off bacterial and viral infections and shield you from arthritis distress. They provide total body invigoration of the vital immune system.

1. *Natural Pain Killer.* The amino acid, tryptophan, is a helpful ally of your immune system to provide pain relief. Tryptophan converts into the neurotransmitter serotonin and makes you more resistant to pain. It helps you feel better because it stimulates your immune system to activate beta-endorphins, your brain's natural pain reliever. Tryptophan may be taken safely under supervision of your health practitioner. It's a food so more desirable than a drug.

2. *Contrast Compresses.* Increase sluggish circulation with the use of alternate hot and cold compresses on the aching area. About 20 minutes each will stimulate production of healing macrophages to destroy invading bacteria.

3. *Say No to Caffeine.* Whether in coffee, tea, soft drinks, chocolate, or medications, it is an enemy of your immune system. Caffeine whips up your adrenal gland to send forth hormones that make you sensitive to pain. Avoid caffeine . . . and you avoid arthritic pain!

4. *Avoid Smoking.* Arthritics who smoke play havoc with the immune system. Nicotine blocks your body's natural pain relievers and your adrenalin glands release hormones to again make you more vulnerable to pain. Keep away from others who smoke, too.

5. *Exercise Is Essential.* Don't just sit there and let your immune system become sedentary! You weaken your muscles and inhibit production of important T-cells needed by your system to fight off arthritic invaders. At least 30 minutes daily of sensible exercise boosts resistance to arthritis and speeds up the healing process.

6. *Ice Away Discomfort.* Freeze water in an empty margarine tub. Rub the aching area in circles for 10 to 15 minutes. Cold numbs, prevents, or reduces swelling. It alerts your immune system to inhibit histamine release which is to blame for pain and inflammation. (*Caution:* If troubled with Raynaud's disease, hypersensitivity to cold, or peripheral vascular disease, ask your health practitioner before trying the ice remedy.)

7. *Keep Regular Hours.* You'll sleep better and awaken with less incidence of morning stiffness with a regular sleep schedule. Erratic sleep patterns can upset your immune rhythm and give you late-night and early-morning aches.

8. *Eat on a Regular Schedule.* Your immune responses function more effectively if you maintain a regular eating schedule. Whether three, five, or six meals daily, follow a comfortable schedule for balanced immune response.

9. *Avoid Irritations.* Constant physical irritations can suppress functions of the immune system. Whether at home or at the workplace (or both), keep such distress signals to a minimum

since they slow immune functions and render you vulnerable to arthritis among other ailments.

10. *Enjoy Refreshing Sleep.* A good night's sleep is the repair shop for your immune system. During rest, this system gathers energy reserves left over from the body's needs during the day to build resistance to infections.

11. *Relax . . . Easy Does It.* Competition, difficulties, and deadlines all lead to stress which depresses your immune system. Haven't you frequently felt arthritis flareup after a stressful situation? When too much pressure builds up, take a walk, a jogging run, or any enjoyable diversion that helps you relieve tension.

12. *Shhhhhh!* Noise can destroy your immune barriers. Your system needs reasonable peace and quiet so it can gather up immune resources and help destroy invading pathogens. Make every effort to shield yourself from excessive noise. How much is too much? If it annoys you!

REBUILDS IMMUNE SYSTEM AND RECOVERS FROM ARTHRITIS IN 30 DAYS

Medications made Janet McM. so sleepy she wondered if the drug was worse than her recurring arthritis. Her limbs were not only stiff but so inflamed she would cry out with pain when anyone touched her. Friends and family kept away from her because she was so edgy. Mornings were difficult. It took her two hours before she could get dressed and prepare meals, and these minor efforts brought stabbing pain spasms to her arms and shoulders. She walked in a hunched-over position. She looked much older than her early 40s. There was no relief in sight.

A nurse at the clinic she visited for treatment suggested she obtain help from an immunologist newly arrived at the facility. Janet McM. tried it with skepticism. A test showed she had a depressed immune system which made her susceptible to arthritic infection. She was given the list of 12 steps to immune invigoration along with a boost in needed nutrients.

Desperate, she followed the program. In two weeks, she could get out of bed with more flexibility. The inflammation cooled. By the third week, she could work around the house with few spasms. By the end of the fourth week, she was as agile as a youngster. "What arthritis?" she asked when she started playing regular tennis with familiar people. The 12 steps had rebuilt her immune system and her T- and B-cells were stabilized as infectious irritants were washed out of her system. She was "as good as new!"

In healing arthritis with a stronger immune system, it is necessary to rebuild the entire body. In some situations, one nutrient is helpful. In others, the spectrum of other nutrients need to be brought into use to strike back at arthritis . . . and win.

IN REVIEW

1. Martha J. overcame "hopeless" arthritis and drugs with a simple doctor's nutritional immune diet program.
2. A noted arthritis specialist has healed thousands with a basic 12-step program that stimulates the immune system and speeds recovery.
3. Yucca extract, available at health stores, is recommended by a physician to ease arthritis pain. This herb also balances blood pressure and cholesterol-triglyceride levels at the same time.
4. Arthritis is linked to a weakness in the immune system. You can correct it with nutritional and other natural therapies right at home.
5. An everyday vitamin has the power to stimulate the T-cells to send forth needed B-cells that will fight arthritic pain-causing invaders in your body.
6. Oscar A. enjoys a simple daily fruit drink that has restored flexibility to his limbs and made him free of pain. The drink bolsters the arthritic-fighting immune system.
7. Invigorate your immune system with a set of 12 simple tricks. Cool inflammation, ease pain, enjoy healthier lifestyle.
8. Janet McM. overcame arthritis in 30 days by rebuilding her immune system with the 12-step plan.

2

Unmasking Arthritis:
What Lies Beneath

A weakness in the complex defense mechanisms your body uses to resist illness and infection is a major reason for your arthritic condition.

Arthritis Invaders

Foreign invaders include pathogens such as viruses, bacteria, fungi, protozoa, parasites, and cellular waste materials. These pain-producing enemies penetrate your immune barrier. Your system retaliates by alerting white blood cells, known as phagocytes, and sends them off to destroy these invaders by engulfing and—literally—eating them. It is important to have a strong defense mechanism to resist the invasion of foreign substances. Nutrition is a major means of building immunity to this threat to your health.

T- and B-Cells Resist Arthritis

A nutritionally sound defense system brings into use the T-lymphocyte cells which are programmed to detect and destroy harmful invaders. The same system uses B-lymphocyte cells to produce antibodies which neutralize and destroy a wider range of these threats to your health.

The T- and B-cells have an extraordinary ability to recognize the exact identity of foreign substances (antigens). Once the arthritic invader has been sighted, the immune response produces substances that defuse and eliminate virally infected cells.

How Immune Cells Cleanse Arthritic Invaders

The T-cells activate the reproduction of B-cells residing in the lymph nodes, which in turn manufacture substances known as antibodies (or immunoglobulins). These substances are complex protein molecules programmed to attack and destroy the arthritic invaders.

Phagocytes travel throughout the infected area, engulfing and "eating" the remains of damaged cells and viral materials, while helper T-cells continue to bring in reinforcements.

When the defense mechanism is over, the last set of T-cells, called suppressor T-cells, begins to release substances which gradually inactivate the entire process, after which the immune response comes to a halt.

The entire process is sparked with energy from nutrition. If there is a deficiency or imbalance, or if your lifestyle is stressful and your emotions are taking their toll, the immune response is either weakened or inadequate. The foreign invaders take hold and arthritis develops.

INTERFERON: KEY TO PAIN RELIEF

Interferon is a protein molecule secreted by T-cells which serves to protect healthy cells from invading pathogens. This substance is able to help protect you from pain. Many have found it to be a natural pain reliever. But when you have weakness in your immune system, there is a reduction of the production of interferon and arthritic pain results.

Your body is able to produce interferon more abundantly so that pain is eased and your immune system is able to wash out hurtful invaders from your system.

A combination of healthy foods, nutritional supplementation, and exercise can enhance the functioning of your body's natural immune systems to boost pain-relieving interferon and create optimal health.

NUTRIENTS THAT BOOST IMMUNE RESPONSE

Several important nutrients are able to stimulate the production of the essential immune fighters, the T- and B-cells and the pain reliever, interferon. These nutrients strengthen your immune system to speed the healing processes and also prevent serious problems. The major immune-nourishing nutrients are:

Vitamin A—needed to produce bacteria-fighting cells in moisture depots of your body. It helps preserve your skin and mucous membranes, important barriers against infection. *Sources:* sweet potato, carrots, squash, broccoli, cantaloupe, mango, apricots, poultry, beef.

Vitamin B-complex—specifically, B2 (riboflavin), B6 (pyridoxine), and pantothenic acid which produce important antibodies to fight off infectious invaders. Also needed is Vitamin B12 to produce T- and B-cells that seek out and ultimately destroy arthritic infections. *Sources:* brewer's yeast, potatoes, salmon, whole grains, mushrooms, cauliflower, broccoli, beef liver.

Vitamin C—stimulates T- and B-cell transformation and is vital in the manufacture of pain-easing interferon. Increased intake of this vitamin greatly enhances phagocytosis, enabling more rapid movement to infected areas and a more efficient destruction of invading arthritis-causing pathogens. *Sources:* oranges, grapefruits, tangerines, guava, strawberries, papaya, green peppers, turnip greens, kale, broccoli, Brussels sprouts, cabbage.

Vitamin E—unique in being able to enhance the production of both antibodies and phagocytes to boost the immune system and manufacture T-cells. *Sources:* cold-processed oils, unrefined foods, wheat germ, green leafy vegetables, nuts, seeds.

Selenium—potentiates phagocytic activity in general and creates a stronger immune barrier. *Sources:* seafood, beef kidney, garlic, mushrooms, whole grains.

Zinc—an important immune-boosting nutrient which is involved in the manufacture of T-cells. *Sources:* wheat germ, wheat bran, cowpeas, cheddar cheese.

These nutrients trigger the immune system to initiate a defensive action to protect you from arthritic and other hurtful invaders. If you plan your daily eating menu to include a variety of the preceding immune-nourishing foods, you should be able to strengthen your system to resist and cast out threats to your well-being.

FROM PAIN TO PEACE IN SIX WEEKS

Eating on the road was common for salesman Lester K. who consumed overcooked and devitalized foods wherever they were available. In his late 40s, he began to develop sore shoulders and low back pain that made driving difficult. At times, he found it hurtful to get up from his seat as a sharp pain made him wince with a low moan. Stiffness limited his movements. There were days when he could hardly bend his back to get out of his car when making a sales call. He feared the onset of arthritis.

A neurologist conducted tests and learned that Lester K.'s body was very deficient in a number of vitamins and some minerals. His immune system was malnourished and infectious invaders threatened the onset of arthritis. A program was outlined in which he not only had to do more physical exercise and avoid stress, but also adjust his eating methods to include more healthful foods.

Lester K. switched to freshly cooked or raw fruits and vegetables, modest amounts of meats, and more whole grains. He soon strengthened his immune system via intake of Vitamin A, B-complex, C, E, and the valuable minerals such as selenium and zinc. These nutrients helped manufacture T-cells and also B-cells which defused arthritis invaders and soon rebuilt his immune system. Within six weeks, his stiff pain had gone. He had youthful flexibility. He happily said his body was peacefully content. He bid arthritis goodbye thanks to a well-nourished immune system.

ARTHRITIS—THE NATION'S MOST COMMON CHRONIC CONDITION

Arthritis strikes one in every seven Americans. It affects people of all ages, including children and adults in the prime of life. This serious health condition affects over 36 million Americans—more than any other chronic condition.

The facts are:

—8.3 million are under 45
—16.1 million are between 45 and 65
—11.6 million are 65 and over
—One in every three families is affected
—Women are affected by arthritis twice as often as men
—$14 billion is the annual cost to the economy in lost wages and medical bills.

What Is Arthritis?

The word arthritis literally means joint inflammation (*arth* = joint; *itis* = inflammation) and refers to more than 100 separate conditions that attack joints and connective tissues. The most common types are the following:

Osteoarthritis

It affects nearly 7 percent of the population and generally results from wear and tear in the mechanical parts of a joint. A weakness in the immune system will affect the weight-bearing joints such as the hips, knees, and ankles. Occupational stress, injuries, overweight, and even heredity predispose to this weakness or suppression of the immune system to open the doorway to osteoarthritis.

Rheumatoid Arthritis

It affects about 1 percent of the population, can begin at any age, but typically occurs between ages 20 and 55. While it can affect the entire body, the joints most commonly involved are those of the hands and feet. A defect in the body's own defense or immune system is a major cause of this condition. (See Figure 2–1.)

THE CAUSE (AND HEALING) OF INFLAMMATION

Inflammation is a reaction of the body that causes swelling, redness, pain, and loss of motion in an affected area. It is the major physical problem in the most serious forms of arthritis.

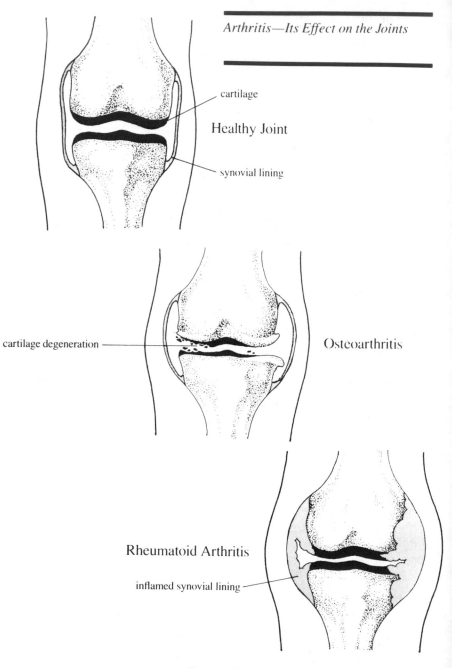

cartilage

Healthy Joint

synovial lining

cartilage degeneration

Osteoarthritis

Rheumatoid Arthritis

inflamed synovial lining

Figure 2–1

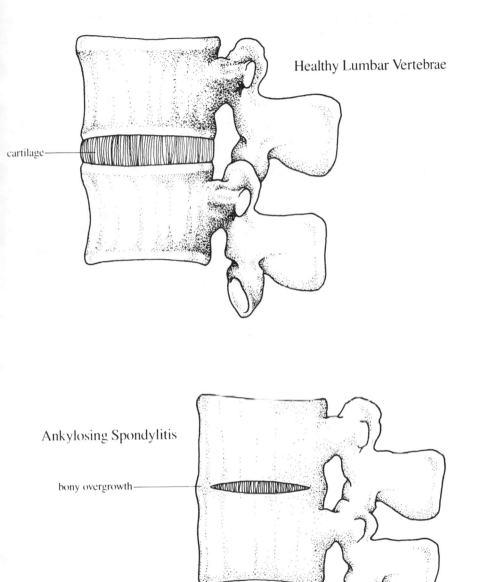

Healthy Lumbar Vertebrae

cartilage

Ankylosing Spondylitis

bony overgrowth

Figure 2–1 (Cont'd.)

Normally, inflammation is the way the body responds to an injury or to the presence of disease agents such as viruses or bacteria. During this reaction, many cells of the body's defense system, called the immune system, rush to the injured area to wipe out the cause of the problem, clean up damaged cells, and repair tissues that have been hurt. Once the "battle" is won, the inflammation normally goes away and the area becomes healthy again.

Immune System Defect

A malnourished or weakened immune system means that the inflammation does not go away as it should. Instead, it becomes part of the problem, damaging healthy tissues of the body. This may result in more inflammation, more damage, and so on in a continuing cycle. The damage that occurs can change the bones and other tissues of the joints, sometimes affecting their shape and making movement hard and painful.

Conditions in which the immune system malfunctions and attacks healthy parts of the body are called autoimmune diseases.

With a stronger immune system, your body is able to uproot and cast out invaders and restore cooling tranquility to your joints and related organs and systems.

SEVEN WARNING SIGNS OF A WEAKENED IMMUNE SYSTEM

1. Swelling in one or more joints.
2. Early-morning stiffness.
3. Recurring pain or tenderness in any joint.
4. Inability to move a joint normally.
5. Obvious redness and warmth in a joint.
6. Unexplained weight loss, fever, or weakness combined with joint pain.
7. Symptoms such as these that last for more than two weeks.

It is important to obtain a correct diagnosis by your health practitioner to confirm which type of arthritis you may have and how to boost your immune responses. The key is in obtaining proper help early in the course of the condition and in faithfully staying with the immune-boosting treatment program even during remissions. That is, you have times when you feel no symptoms. There are other times when the condition gets worse and flares. It is this see-saw reaction that should alert you to continue with your immune strengthening program until you have been diagnosed as "out of danger."

A DISORDER OF THE IMMUNE SYSTEM

Molecular biologists have noted that a malfunction of the immune system is responsible for many situations of joint inflammation and the hurt of arthritis.

The triggering agents include viruses; bacteria (or components of bacterial cell walls); collagen, the normal scaffolding or supporting structure found in all connective tissues of the body; and, of course, even one of the body's own immune defenders, specifically the antibody immunoglobulin IgG, also known as gamma globulin. Note that only two of these possible causes—viruses and bacteria—are external agents.

Is It Genetic?

A malfunction of the immune system is often said to be genetically determined. This does not mean the condition is handed down from one generation to the next. It means that genetic factors control the mode and intensity of the immune response.

INFLAMMATION, IMMUNE SYSTEM, INTERNAL STRUGGLE

In rheumatoid arthritis, for example, the difficulty begins when the immune system encounters an unknown foreign substance or "non-self"; i.e., an antigen. Even at an early stage, the immunologic battle may not be localized at the joint. You may be systemically ill with non-specific symptoms of low-grade fever, malaise, and fatigue. Some early stages of arthritis mimic that of an infectious disease such as influenza.

Trouble Within Your Body

The monocyte, one of the white blood cells, is the cell to first recognize the antigen. When the monocytes encounter something they perceive as foreign, they go into action and conduct an internal chemical warfare against it. They "process" the antigen, present it to antigen-specific T-lymphocytes, which produce antibodies that combine only with that antigen.

These complexes of antigen and antibody are removed by phagocytes, the polymorphonuclear cells, that literally eat the antigen-antibody combinations. In doing so, they regurgitate enzymes and generate other products which cause inflammation. These substances also attack body tissues and produce chemicals that attract even more phagocytes into the joint space.

Reason for the Hurt

Phagocytosis also activates systems which produce prostaglandins and leukotrienes. *Problem:* the prostaglandins may stimulate pain and cause capillaries within the joint to dilate and become leaky. As a consequence, blood rushes into the area while lymphocytes and phagocytes leak out into the tissues. The joint becomes hot, swollen, and painful. Leukotrienes are chemotactic; that is, they act as a biological magnet to draw more phagocytic cells into the joint cavity.

Malnourished Immune System Is Self-Destructive

With a malnourished immune system, the inflammatory ferment within the joint runs wild. Cells in the joint lining are threatened. Some chemicals released make the synovial cells (needed to provide lubrication for movement) divide and re-divide very quickly. The synovium (fine membrane lining the joint) situated at the periphery of the joint is transformed into a thick, coarse cell mass called pannus. The pannus proliferates inward, toward the center of the joint, destroying cartilage and bone as it advances by producing enzymes that dissolve the cartilage.

If unchecked, this self-destructive reaction could destroy the cartilage. The pannus retreats. The inflammation recedes.

This leaves a ruined joint without cartilage and without normal function. The body tends to self-destruct, so to speak.

NUTRITIONAL IMMUNITY: BARRIER AGAINST ARTHRITIS

Scientists feel one key to treating arthritis is to strengthen the immune system, to find nutritional techniques that cool inflammation, and to establish equilibrium within the body to protect against self-destruction.

In some situations, a single nutrient or food helps plug the gap in the fortress of immunity. In other cases, a total nutritional plan is required to strengthen the immune system and cast out offending invaders. It is important to cooperate with your health practitioner. Your goal should be a total body makeover to be free of arthritis via a strong immune system.

SIX STEPS TO COOLING-HEALING RHEUMATOID ARTHRITIS

A defect in the immune system could trigger an invasion of harmful substances that lead to joint inflammation along with painful swelling. Since rheumatoid arthritis affects the entire body, it is important to use a holistic approach in cooling and healing the disorder. To stimulate a sluggish immune system for holistic recovery, here is a basic six-step program easily followed by everyone:

1. *Protein Power.* Protein acts as building blocks of the body, you need protein to nourish your immune system and restore a strong barrier against infectious invaders. Protein also gives vigor to processes that cast out hurtful elements. This immune food is found in lean meats, fish, egg whites, dairy products, peas, beans, nuts, and also as protein powders available in nutrition centers. Aim for at least 40 grams of protein daily, or one generous serving.

2. *Calcium Is Cooling.* Calcium helps the damaged joints repair themselves and cools off painful areas. Cartilage is also nourished by calcium (and protein). This immune mineral is

Major Forms of Arthritis

	Incidence in U.S.	Symptoms	Prognosis
Osteoarthritis	17 million, mostly elderly. More common in women. Seen in younger patients following joint injury.	Pain, loss of mobility in one or more joints.	Progressive joint deterioration if untreated. May be halted by prescribed rest, exercise, and medication.
Rheumatoid Arthritis	7 million. Often strikes between ages 20 and 45. Women victims outnumber men three to one.	Symmetric joint pain, swelling, and possible deformity; morning stiffness; fatigue; weight loss.	Chronic degenerative disease with periodic remissions. May be crippling if not treated promptly with program of medication, rest, exercise, and other therapy.
Juvenile Rheumatoid Arthritis	250,000 children. May begin before age seven.	Knee or other joint pain and stiffness. Sometimes starts with high fever, rash, and no joint symptoms.	Can cause eye inflammation, growth abnormalities. Treatment generally prevents damage. Seventy percent outgrow the disease with no residual effects.

Disease	Incidence	Symptoms	Course/Treatment
Ankylosing Spondylosis	2.5 million. Seems more common in males. Appears as early as teens or 20s.	Pain and stiffness in spine.	Progressive spinal curvature and loss of spinal mobility. Generally controlled by medication, postural training, and exercise.
Gout	1.6 million. Most victims male. Generally strikes after age 40.	Sudden onset of acute pain and inflammation usually in a single joint—often big toe.	Joint damage prevented and recurrence controlled by medication and diet.
Scleroderma	300,000 victims. Most women in their 40s and 50s.	Tightness or hardening of skin. Often affects joints and internal organs.	May progress rapidly or become chronic. Treatment rarely completely successful.
Systemic Lupus Erythematosus	300,000 victims. Approximately 10 females for every male. Incidence higher in blacks. First appearance anytime from teens to 50s.	May start with fever, weakness, weight loss, and rash, particularly on arms, neck, and face. Joint pain and symptoms of organ damage may follow.	Course of disease depends on amount of internal organ involvement. Five-year survival with treatment now exceeds 90 percent.

—Courtesy of the Upjohn Company

25

found in skim milk products, brewer's yeast, dandelion greens, salmon or sardines canned with bones, yogurt, mustard greens, almonds, broccoli. Supplements are also available.

3. *Seafood Is Important.* Fish contains *eicosapentaenoic acid* (EPA) and *docosabexaenoic acid* (DHA), which have been shown to reduce inflammation and ease morning stiffness and pain. Eat fish as often as possible to bolster your immune system and help cool off inflammation and pain.

4. *Lose Weight.* If you have arthritis in weight-bearing joints, such as the knees and hips, excess weight imposes stress and worsens the pain. Joints will also deteriorate more quickly. Don't overload your immune system with overweight. Reduce and you also reduce symptoms and give your immune network the ability to provide protection without being burdened down.

5. *Avoid Stress.* Tension of any sort weakens your immune system and triggers flareups. Other conditions that influence stress are overexertion, improper rest, changes in familiar routine, family illness, and work or money difficulties. A happier disposition and lifestyle maintains a stronger immune system and less arthritic distress.

6. *Keep Active.* Your immune system reacts joyfully when you are fit. Whether you walk, jog, swim, bicycle, or work out, your joints have to be kept mobile through moderate and regular exercise. *Careful:* Too much exercise may be painful. Try stretching, isometrics (yoga, for example), swimming, where body weight is supported.

Build this six-step program into your lifestyle and your immune system will be invigorated to help you cope and cast out arthritis invaders from your body . . . and mind.

FIGHTS AND WINS ARTHRITIS BATTLE

Barbara DeG. first encountered rheumatoid arthritis when she found it difficult to put on makeup in the morning. Her fingers on both hands were stiff and awkward. Over the next few months, pain and swelling developed. Mornings were very hurtful, and not until noon did she have some flexibility, although the pain caused her to wince when she tried to grasp a utensil or pick up the telephone.

Medications relieved the disorder to some extent but Barbara DeG. felt dizzying side effects and stomach upset. She was examined by a medical nutritionist who diagnosed her as being deficient in a number of important nutrients. The prescribed medications had induced a "washout" of the nutrients she needed to strengthen the immune system to resist arthritis.

Barbara DeG. followed the preceding six-step plan and supervised medication adjustment. Withdrawal symptoms were uncomfortable but gradually, she felt her stiffness subsiding and the inflammation cooling off. Swelling went down, too. After 60 days, she felt "as good as new" thanks to a stronger immune system. The nutritional and fitness program had helped her fight (and win) against arthritis!

OVERCOME OSTEOARTHRITIS WITH AN INVIGORATED IMMUNE SYSTEM

"Wear and tear" is often said to lead to this type of arthritis. The immune system is unable to cope with demands upon the body. Cartilage between the surfaces of connected bones usually provides a cushion between the two joints. A defect in the immune system means the cartilage's ability to self-repair cannot keep pace with the degeneration it goes through during daily use. If the cartilage wears away, the two connecting bones will grate upon one another. Joints could become swollen, inflamed, and misshapen. Osteoarthritis sets in.

Problem: Prescribed and over-the-counter drugs will drain out nutrients from your body. A thorough diagnosis is needed to determine any of your possible deficiencies. Typical losses from most drugs are: Vitamin C, folic acid, and iron. Supplementation as prescribed will help make up for this loss and strengthen the immune system.

To stimulate your immune system and help ease and erase osteoarthritic symptoms, this simple program is easily followed:

1. Lose excess weight. Surplus poundage puts hurtful pressure on weight-bearing joints and this weakens your immune

system which worsens the arthritis. A lean body is a picture of a stronger immune system.

2. Both calcium and protein should be consumed daily so your immune system is able to keep your cartilage and bone in a healthy state.

3. There is much evidence to suggest that fish oils contain ingredients that help prevent and cool inflammatory reactions in the body. Eat seafood regularly to bolster your immune system's ability to protect against osteoarthritic symptoms.

4. Wake up your sluggish immune system with regular exercise. For osteoarthritis, isometrics help maintain muscle tone and strengthen them. Isometrics are those in which the muscle is tensed without causing motion at the joints. (Yoga, for example.) Isotonics are hurtful and may damage the joints so should be avoided for osteoarthritics. Isotonics maintain uniform muscle tone but cause movement at the joints such as in fast running. *Plan:* About 15 to 30 minutes a day sets off a better flow of T-lymphocytes and B-lymphocytes to activate antibodies that will cast out arthritic invaders.

5. Try a warm soak or hot pack to relieve tightness and pain in the muscle, because the warmth helps send forth soothing antibodies via your immune system to the site of discomfort. Apply comfortable warmth twice a day for 15 to 30 minutes in order for your immune system to react.

The preceding five-step program alerts your immune system to start defensive action and cleanse away harmful invaders responsible for discomfort.

SAVED FROM "HOPELESS" OSTEOARTHRITIS IN THREE WEEKS

Michael R. V. was told he was "burned out" on his job. He was only 49 and already a company supervisor with a vice-presidency almost within reach. What was wrong? He had stiff joints, felt understandably depressed, and winced because of swollen fingers.

Several retired former co-workers who also had osteoarthritis said his condition was "hopeless" and to "give up." Michael

R. V. refused. He had a thorough examination by an endocrinologist and nutritional specialist. The report revealed nutritional deficiencies brought on by constant drug use. He was overweight. He was sedentary and had let himself "slide" in terms of fitness.

He was put on a nutritional program to make up for drug-induced lost nutrients. Weight loss and fitness combined with warm soaks helped bolster his immune system in a short time.

Within 20 days, he no longer felt restrictive stiffness or swelling pain. He joined a company bowling team and became a winner . . . as well as a V-P. "Burn out?" he laughed. "We've just begun . . . my immune system and I."

You, too, can rebuild your life and free yourself from the ravages of arthritis with a stronger immune system. The key to recovery is a nutritional and total body makeover plan. Rebuild your immune system and you have a "miracle cure" within your own body!

IN REVIEW

1. Newer scientific discoveries link arthritis to breaks in the immune system.
2. Boost T- and B-lymphocyte production to ease pain with the use of vitamin-rich foods.
3. Lester K. overcame threatening arthritis with a simple immune-boosting nutritional plan easily followed anywhere.
4. Note the workings of the immune system as a protective barrier, and the warning signs of arthritis.
5. A six-step program helps cool and heal rheumatoid arthritis in a short time.
6. Barbara DeG. became reborn and freed of arthritis by following the "miracle" six-step immune-boosting program.
7. Overcome osteoarthritis with a five-step immune-strengthening plan.
8. Michael R. V. overcame "hopeless" osteoarthritis in three weeks with a simple body makeover program. His stimulated immune system gave him a brand-new, healthy, arthritis-free future!

3

The "No-Nightshade" Diet Says Goodbye to Arthritis

Clinical evidence exists that allergy is the major cause of arthritis in many people. Rheumatologists explain that arthritics have become allergic to themselves. This is the reason that rheumatoid arthritis, for example, is often called an autoimmune condition. Newer research in immunology has isolated many blood factors which support this discovery.

THE FOOD GROUP THAT UPSETS THE IMMUNE BARRIER

"Food allergies are a major problem in 50 percent of people with arthritis, compared with only 5 percent of allergy to foods in otherwise healthy persons," says Robert Bingham, M.D., of the Desert Arthritis Medical Clinic of Desert Hot Springs, California.

"Arthritis is one of the conditions which is triggered by an allergic reaction to the nightshade family of plants." These foods contain *solanine,* a toxic substance that penetrates the immune barrier and creates a painful reaction.

Nightshades, Allergy, Arthritis Outbreak

In many arthritics, the solanine is a threat and the body's immune system attacks it as an allergic invader. As soon as solanine penetrates the immune barrier, the body reacts by

31

making large amounts of an immunoglobulin antibody. These IgE molecules want to uproot and cast out this invader. They do so by attaching to the surfaces of mast cells or basophil. This is a special white blood cell, also called a granulocyte. It is filled with granules of protective substances that can digest the solanine microorganisms and render them harmless.

When the IgE molecules or antibodies, sitting on the mast cell or basophil, encounter their specific solanine microorganisms, the IgE antibodies signal to the mast cell to release the powerful substances inside it. These are the mediators that cause the allergic symptoms of your arthritis. You feel aches, stiffness, often agonizing pain because of this inner immune response.

Dr. Bingham comments, "The solanine-containing 'nightshade' foods are highly toxic to many arthritis patients, especially when consumed over a period of months or years.

"Solanines may be the only cause of arthritis in some patients; in others, a secondary cause that interferes with their recovery."

FOUR FOODS AND ONE PLANT WHICH MAY CAUSE ARTHRITIS

The solanine-containing foods which may be toxic in many arthritic patients are:

1. White potatoes—*solanum tuberosum*
2. Eggplant—*solanum melongena*
3. Tomatoes—*lycopersicum esculenium*
4. Red peppers—*capsicum ssp.*
Plant: Tobacco—*solanaceae*

The most common early symptoms are pain and joint stiffness. An elimination diet will disclose the offending foods and alert you to this allergic reaction. If you eliminate these four foods and tobacco in all forms, your immune system will help protect you from the painful allergy of an antibody alert.

THOUSANDS HEALED ON "NO-NIGHTSHADE" DIET

Norman F. Childers, Ph.D., Professor of Horticulture at the University of Florida, tells of being stricken with severe arthritis. After reading that cattle grazing on plants of the nightshade family developed severe arthritic pain, he self-experimented by withdrawing these foods from his own diet. He achieved complete relief from his arthritis.

Victory Over Arthritis

Dr. Childers organized a group of "cooperators"—thousands of individuals with arthritis who were willing to experimentally withdraw these foods from their diets. A large number of them became partially or totally relieved of their stiffness, aches, pains, and restricted joint mobility.

When many of these people were bold enough to try eating nightshade plants again, they experienced a defect in their immune systems and a painful return of arthritic complications. The conclusion was announced: eliminate nightshades and you may well eliminate arthritis and become victorious in the battle.

WHEELCHAIR ARTHRITICS RECOVER

In some instances, people were so badly crippled by arthritis they had to be confined to bed, or use walkers and wheelchairs. On the "no-nightshade" diet, they reported benefits ranging from relief to total recovery!

STIFF ARTHRITIC FINGER BECOMES FLEXIBLE

Professor John L. told Dr. Childers, "Originally, I was totally resistant to these findings. It looks as if I am beginning to weaken a bit relative to the effects of nightshade plants on many people with arthritis.

"Last summer, I eliminated these particular vegetables from my diet. Previously, for a year, the little finger of my right hand was badly afflicted—I could not open it when arising in the morning without assistance.

"Since early last November that trouble has entirely disappeared. Why? I don't know, but it looks as if the variations in diet, the elimination of the nightshades, could well have been responsible. I hope so."[1]

---

[1] Norman F. Childers, Ph.D., "A Diet to Stop Arthritis," University of Florida.

It should be emphasized that Dr. Childers does not blame all cases of arthritis on eating the nightshade vegetables. He is addressing himself to what amounts to an allergic reaction in some arthritics. The gradual intake of the toxic substance, solanine, might be responsible for a breakdown in immune response. It is easy to drop these foods and see if you have a benefit for your aches and pains. At least you will not be toying with the side reactions of aspirins, corticosteroids, and anti-inflammation drugs.

FROM "BENT OVER WITH A CANE" TO ATHLETIC FIGURE WITHIN WEEKS ON "NO-NIGHTSHADE" DIET

Joe V. was so crippled with arthritis, he had to walk with a cane. He had tried different remedies to no avail. He was told of the "no nightshade" diet by his rheumatologist and decided to try it since he had "nothing to lose but the pain."

Within a very short time, a number of weeks, he walked easily, a straight figure and without any cane. By omitting the taboo foods from his diet as well as ending his tobacco habit, he was able to strengthen his immune system and resist the arthritic symptoms caused by solanine.

Hidden Sources of Nightshades

Avoiding this group of antagonistic foods requires a bit of extra care. For example, some yogurt contains enough potato starch (needed to give the product a thick consistency) to cause arthritic pain to flare. Chocolate may sometimes interfere with the immune system when you follow the diet. Packaged foods may contain white potato and tomato products. Some cheeses contain paprika (derived from peppers) and those cheeses with a pink color may also contain pepper. It is important to read labels of all processed foods to determine if they contain hidden sources of nightshades.

OVERCOMES CRIPPLING ARTHRITIS IN FIVE WEEKS

In a reported situation, a 60-year-old man had osteoarthritis, said to be "the worst case we've seen in years." He had to be helped from bed in the morning, and was placed between two vertical boards, which were then strapped tightly around him, enabling him for short periods to stand erect at the price of considerable pain.

Leo O'C. was put on the "no-nightshade" diet and also given large doses of niacinamide (Vitamin B3). Before long, he was able to pursue normal activity although he still has a slight degree of pain in the hip area. Within five weeks, he no longer needed the boards or other appliances and could pursue normal activities. His immune system had been strengthened to resist allergic reactions because he eliminated the solanine-containing foods.[2]

MEDICAL REPORTS OF SUCCESS ON "NO-NIGHTSHADE" DIET

Dr. Robert Bingham gives examples from medical colleagues who have been able to strengthen the immune system in patients and heal arthritis:

*A 58-year-old male had undergone conventional therapy for synovitis and was walking on crutches due to a painful, swollen knee. With correction of his allergies, he recovered and "has remained free of arthritis for the past seven years, playing golf and tennis and running daily."

*When 127 arthritic patients were given corrective diet, there was a 59 percent success rate in relieving all painful symptoms because of a stronger and resistant immune system.

*Several patients told of being "sensitive" to certain foods. The physician put them on a special diet and reported a healing because "food sensitivity brought on rheumatoid arthritis."

*Another physician described by Dr. Bingham "claims to have cured thousands of arthritics with a fixed low-allergen diet."

*Still another physician, Dr. T. G. Randolph, summarized his 25-year experience with over 200 rheumatoid arthritis cases by noting they could favorably respond to allergy treatment "with but rare exceptions." Indeed, most of the clinical evidence

---

[2] *Prevention Magazine,* April, 1983, p. 30.

demonstrates a clear cause-and-effect relationship between foods eaten and arthritic pain.[3]

MORE PROOF OF ARTHRITIS HEALING ON "NO-NIGHTSHADE" DIET

Dr. Bingham notes that in over 232 cases from four independent investigators, the following observations were made:

1. Acute arthritic symptoms disappeared following a restricted (or fasting) diet for five to seven days.
2. Symptoms recurred when certain nightshade foods were individually restored to the diet.
3. Symptoms disappeared again when each such food was withdrawn.
4. Most patients experienced several cycles of symptom production and remission in response to foods.
5. No regression was observed when patients continued with normal diets from which only the offending foods were eliminated (except when a patient injudiciously ate an allergenic food.)

It is also reported that nightshade allergy symptoms typically exacerbate during the night or early morning, perhaps accounting for arthritic morning stiffness.

The solanine-containing nightshade foods are highly toxic to many arthritis patients, especially when consumed over a period of months or years.

LITTLE-KNOWN SOURCES OF IMMUNE-DESTROYING NIGHTSHADES

The large nightshade family of plants *(solanaceae)* native to tropical America is one of the leading sources of foods, drugs, and ornamental plants. The typical sources include white potato, eggplant, tomatoes, and red peppers.

---

[3] T. G. Randolph, M.D., *Clinical Ecology.* C.C. Thomas Publishing Co., Springfield, Illinois, 1976.

Lesser known sources are ground cherries as well as any nicotine-containing product. Tobacco is a concentrated source of solanin.

Drugs include nicotine (from *nicotiana*), belladonna and atropine (from *atropa*), henbane (from *hyoscyamus*), and stramonium (from *datura*).

Certain of these plants, however, contain toxic chemicals that cause illness, even death, in humans and animals when ingested in quantities above the "safe level," including the highly toxic nightshades.

The origin of the term "nightshades" may be their "evil and loving nature of the night," according to ancient lore. The Romans in the old days were said to prepare potions of the deadly nightshades and offer them to their enemies. While these are extremes, it indicates some people could have a weakness in the immune system that will react when solanine-containing foods are consumed.

With this view, the nutritional approach suggests that no arthritic patient can be considered completely and thoroughly treated without a trial on the "no nightshades" diet. Although these foods probably add up to only 10 percent of the average diet, they play such a large role in the typical food program, it is often difficult to reduce or eliminate them. Yet studies reportedly indicate that *more than half* of arthritis patients suffer some toxic effects from nightshades in either the cause or worsening of their condition.

HOW SOLANINE HURTS THE IMMUNE SYSTEM

The nightshade plants contain a saponic-like glycoalkaloid, an irritant causing red blood cell destruction. They also have a toxic steroid alkamine which is absorbed through the intestine and responsible for the sensitivity symptoms of arthritis.

Checklist of Symptoms

When solanine is absorbed into the body in quantity, it causes anorexia (loss of appetite), nausea, dizziness, abdominal pain, vomiting, constipation or diarrhea (sometimes with blood), anemia, weakness, and accumulation of fluid in the abdomen.

Inflammation can occur in the gastrointestinal tract with ulceration, hemorrhage, and diverticulitis. Cases of acute poisoning are rare but can contribute to the death of the weak or elderly.

Emotional Reactions

Nervous effects from solanine include apathy, drowsiness, salivation, difficulty in breathing, trembling, progressive weakness to the extent of paralysis, and collapse.

Solanine and Arthritis

The most common effects of chronic or low-level solanine poisoning are pain and stiffness. It can occur in many joints, their related muscles and tendons, with joint swelling and skin rash.

Solanine is an inhibitor of cholinesterase, an enzyme that provides agility of muscle movements. If solanine wears down the immune system and causes a depletion of this enzyme, the effect is that of stiffness and slow muscle movement. Joint pain swelling and stiffness attributed to arthritis can be traced to the solanine battle with the immunoglobulin antibodies which try to cast out this foreign invader.

Many arthritics who were diagnosed as having "chronic" or "multiple" symptoms may recover promptly by successfully eliminating the nightshades from their diet.

Simple Self-Test

If you detect a flareup after eating any or all of the nightshade foods, try a simple elimination self-test. Stay away from one or all of the foods for at least two weeks. Then eat the suspect food at least twice in a 24-hour period. The first thing to look for is this: Did your arthritis clear up or improve during the two-week "vacation"? If so, then the second question is: Did your arthritis get worse after the food was again eaten? You can then be guided toward corrective dietary healing and strengthening of the immune system to resist allergic attacks of arthritis.

Of course, any arthritic may have more than one trigger food (and many do), so it would be important to obtain food allergy testing by your medical practitioner.

POTATO—*SOLANUM TUBEROSUM*

The white potato is the most common of the nightshade foods. It originates from Peru and has been used as human food for about 400 years. Glycoalkaloid and solanine can be found throughout the potato, with the most concentration in the peel.

Farmers have found that cattle and horses eating potato vines frequently become ill, develop nervous symptoms and paralysis, and may even die. These toxic reactions are known to growers who attempt to keep the solanine content below 20 mg/100 gm of fresh potatoes, which is thought to be safe for human consumption.

The white potato may provide a calming effect within an hour after eating; then aches set in within the next day or so.

Caution: Besides being eaten whole as a staple in the diet of many people, potatoes are also processed into many prepared foods. Potato products and potato starch are found in baby foods, inexpensive yogurts, gravies, and sauces.

It is interesting to note that when first introduced into Europe by 16th century Spanish explorers, potatoes were at first shunned as food because many thought they were poisonous.

EGGPLANT—*SOLANUM MELONGENA*

Less popular, the eggplant has been used for food only in the present century. In certain countries bordering the Mediterranean, it was thought to cause emotional upset if eaten daily for as long as a month.

Certain European countries have traditionally avoided eggplant because of the arthritic-like responses noted, although there is a gradual acceptance of this vegetable since not everyone is similarly affected.

TOMATO—*LYCOPERSICUM ESCULENTUM*

An excellent source of Vitamins A and C and many minerals, the tomato is an important food. Yet it does have solanine content and could weaken your immune system to bring on arthritic disorders.

In the United States, the tomato was considered poisonous until the early 1800s when a daring government official ate it in public with no ill effects. It has since become a dietary staple. This person was fortunate in that his immune system could resist solanine. Others may not have that strong an immune barrier.

Besides its use as a fresh food, tomatoes are found in many processed foods for flavoring such as sauces, vegetable juices, canned and frozen products, baby foods, and other prepared items.

Tomato vines are poisonous to livestock. Just handling tomatoes or their vines will cause sore, inflamed hands in some people.

RED PEPPER—*CAPSICUM SPP*

Three main varieties of red peppers contain solanines: the sweet or bell pepper; paprika or pimiento; and chili or cayenne pepper.

Safe for use are the black-and-white peppers of the *piperaceae* family which are commonly used as table seasonings.

Chili peppers often used in Hispanic-style food contain solanines that can irritate the gastrointestinal tract, cause skin rash, and reportedly may contribute to the development of arthritis. When the immune system sends forth an outpouring of immunoglobulin antibodies to attach to the cells and neutralize the solanine invaders, the arthritic symptoms are felt: tingling in the chest area, discomfort in arms and legs, and pain settling in different joints at different times.

Hidden sources of red pepper could be cough lozenges, pain-relieving ointments, "hot" gravies and sauces, barbecue sauces, and certain medications which contain its oil.

TOBACCO—*SOLANACEAE*

Also identified as *nicotiana tabacum,* the harmful effects of nicotine are well-known but few are aware of its toxic solanine content. Smoking could be called a "double whammy," injuring arthritic persons in two ways. First, the constant threat of respiratory and cancer disorders; second, the injury performed to the immune system and the eruption of antibody irritation.

It is advisable to avoid smoking—whether your own or inhalation of others in your midst.

ARTHRITIS—IS IT AN ALLERGY?

New research indicates arthritis may well be an allergic reaction to one or more of the nightshade foods. The solanine content has a toxic reaction that leads to symptoms. The immune system subsequently becomes weakened, unable to cope with the solanine accumulation.

By eliminating the nightshade foods, your immune system is able to create greater resistance to the reactions triggered by infectious invaders. You may then enjoy a natural remission of symptoms.

Are you allergic to nightshade foods? Eliminate them. Self-test to see if your symptoms subside and go away. If so, your immune system has become strong enough to cast out the invaders and help you recover from "hopeless" arthritis. The "no nightshade" immune-building program has helped tens of thousands so far. It may well help you enjoy immunity to arthritis.

IN REVIEW

1. Arthritis may be a symptom of an allergic reaction to the nightshade family of plants.
2. A noted professor has seen thousands of arthritics become healed on a simple but amazingly effective "no nightshade" nutritional plan.
3. John L. corrected a stiff finger on the easy nutritional plan in a short time.

4. Joe V. was bent over and had to walk with a cane. His crippling arthritis ended after following the "no nightshade" diet and no smoking.

5. Crippling osteoarthritis confined Leo O'C. to vertical boards or else he could not stand. He followed the immune-building, nightshade-free plan and his immune system was strengthened within five weeks. He overcame the arthritis allergy and was free of splints and pain.

6. Four foods can easily be eliminated as a means of strengthening the immune system to resist toxic invasion of solanine. You can ease and erase arthritis when you omit these foods.

4

The Miracle Vitamin That Lubricates Your Arthritic Joints

One of the first vitamins to receive mention in the treatment of arthritis was niacinamide or Vitamin B3. Medical specialists and pioneers in immunology discovered that the rheumatoid arthritic had a disorder of the T-cells. A reduction in the amount of available phagocytes created a sensitivity to irritants that led to stiffness and painful movements of the joints.

Niacinamide Provides Lubrication

Immunologists report that the rheumatoid arthritic loses far more tryptophan (natural pain killer) than non-arthritics do, thereby creating a deficiency of niacinamide. It was observed that when arthritics took additional amounts of niacinamide, the immune system was stimulated and there was greater retention of tryptophan. Arthritics had reduced pain but even more important to many, the formerly stiff fingers and joints were now more flexible. Niacinamide had acted as a natural lubricant!

Cools Inflamed Joints

Niacinamide mobilizes arachidonic acid (a fatty acid) and stimulates the formation of substances called prostaglandins, some of which combat inflammation.

By including niacinamide, you will be providing power to your phagocytes to "devour" the toxic elements that have penetrated your immune barrier. Niacinamide prompts the phagocytes to give the immunologic barrier much of its vigor in sighting and destroying the foreign invaders. Niacinamide also prompts the macrophages or backup cells to wipe out the harmful substances missed by the others and to create inner cleansing of irritants.

This process enables your immune system to protect your joints from the hurtful and restrictive microorganisms responsible for inflammation and stiffness.

NIACINAMIDE HELPS PREVENT FALLS IN AGING

Because of joint stiffness, many an older arthritic is prone to swaying and falling. It is believed that a weak immune system has disturbed message centers in the brain. That is, the brain no longer receives proper information concerning the position of the arms and legs in movement because of gradual impairment of nerve function.

The T-cell lymphocytes are unable to clear away debris which causes cellular malfunction. The brain is less efficient in perceiving and combining the neural messages coming from the limbs. All of this contributes to the tendency of the elderly to fall more frequently as they age, especially if joint stiffness compounds the problem with less flexibility.

Niacinamide reportedly will help provide more tryptophan which not only acts to ease distress and provide pain-free flexibility but helps to diminish the impact of aging on the sense of balance and muscle tone.

NIACINAMIDE VS. NIACIN: WHICH IS MORE BENEFICIAL?

Essentially, there is no difference between these two available forms of B3. They may be used interchangeably. However, niacin can cause a flushing reaction in some arthritics, characterized by a redness in the face, neck, and other areas, accompanied in many cases by itching. This usually disappears in about a half hour.

If you experience this sensation, switch to a supplement containing niacinamide; it does not cause flushing. The joint lubrication effects will be the same with either variety.

How Much to Take?

The official U.S. Recommended Daily Amount or RDA calls for 20 milligrams. The maximum is said to be 50 milligrams per day. But for an arthritic with a weakened immune system, a boosted amount could be required to help stimulate the needed T-cells which help rid your body of ailing cells. It has been reported that approximately 100 milligrams of niacinamide daily will help relieve much pain and stiffness. You may also benefit from the whole B-complex family of vitamins since they do interact and work together to invigorate your body's defenses and powers of recuperation from arthritic joint stiffness.

Foods That Provide Niacin

Food	Amount (1 portion)	Milligrams
BREAD GROUP		
Wheat bran	⅓ cup	8.3
Wheat germ	¼ cup	2.1
Wheat, shredded	1 biscuit	1.3
Whole wheat bread	1 slice	1.4
Rice, brown, cooked	½ cup	1.2
Lima beans, cooked	⅓ cup	1.7
Soya beans, cooked	⅔ cup	3.6
Potato, baked	1 medium	1.7
MILK GROUP		
Skim milk	8 ounces	2.3
VEGETABLE GROUP		
Mushrooms, raw	10 small or 4 large	4.3
Peas, green, cooked	½ cup	2.5
Broccoli, cooked	1 stalk	1.4
Brussels sprouts, cooked	5–6	1.0

Food	Amount (1 portion)	Milligrams
Corn, cooked	½ ear	1.0
Cucumbers	½ medium	1.0

FRUIT GROUP

Cantaloupe	¼ melon	1.0
Peach	1 medium	.9

MEAT GROUP

Liver	1 ounce	6.9
Tuna	i ounce	5.0
Halibut	1 ounce	3.7
Chicken	1 ounce	3.6
Turkey	1 ounce	3.2
Salmon	1 ounce	3.1
Beef, lamb	1 ounce	3.1
Egg	1 medium	1.7

FAT GROUP

Avocado	⅛ (4-inch diameter)	.5
Peanuts	6 small	1.4

Nourish your immune system with a variety of these niacinamide-containing foods. You will then help cast out infectious invaders that are causing joint stiffness and arthritic distress.

MORNING ARTHRITIS TONIC FOR YOUTHFUL FLEXIBILITY

To boost your immune system with niacinamide from foods, try a tasty and invigorating Morning Arthritis Tonic.

How to Make: 1 cup skim milk combined with 4 tablespoons of wheat bran and 2 pitted peaches may be blenderized and then sipped slowly in the morning.

Benefits: The Morning Arthritis Tonic is a powerful source of concentrated niacinamide with additional B-complex vitamins as well as various minerals. The nutrients work speedily to send forth a supply of tryptophan to help promote greater flexibility of joint motion and a reduction in discomfort. The nutrients stimulate the production of gamma globulin, the kind of protein of which antibodies are made, and thereby strengthen your immune system to destroy any stiffness-causing intruder, such as a bacterium. Joints will soon feel more flexible and able to respond to your needs.

BECOMES YOUTHFULLY FLEXIBLE IN ONE DAY

Anna E. took "forever" to get out of bed in the morning. Her arms were so stiff, she could scarcely button her clothes or lace her shoes. Anna E. felt her arthritis worsening with each step of the way. Not until noontime could she manage to straighten up and attend to her daily chores. She worried about becoming an invalid if the condition worsened.

Drugs offered temporary relief. The side effects were often so distressing, she could not continue with the medication.

Her rheumatologist tested Anna E. to come up with a laboratory report that she was deficient in Vitamin B3. He suggested she take the Morning Arthritis Tonic, reportedly a powerful stimulant to the immune system and helpful in alerting the cellular defenses in dealing with infectious invaders.

From the very start, Anna E. felt a strengthening of her immune system so that she could easily slide out of bed, dress easily, and perform activities with much more youthful flexibility. She was able to boost the tryptophan flow to give her more agility with less discomfort. Niacinamide in the Morning Arthritis Tonic had restored youthful flexibility within one day. She calls it her "get up and go" tonic and "wouldn't be without it for a single day."

ARTHRITIS: IS IT A NUTRITIONAL DEFICIENCY?

In order to adequately determine any nutritional deficiencies and take steps to correct them, laboratory analysis is essential. Routine physical examinations usually reveal the nature and extent of the condition, but laboratory tests supervised by a medical nutritionist will show whether the arthritis is acute or chronic, arrested or spreading, improving or becoming worse, and the nutritional relationship.

The type and degree of dietary deficiency in the arthritic's body can be determined by means of a detailed nutritional analysis. As part of your routine examination, have a dietary analysis made at the same time to reveal any inadequacies.

IMMUNOLOGIC MEDICINE HEALS ARTHRITIC DISORDERS

The newer science of immunology has led to the medical practice of immunology—use of knowledge about the immune system to prevent, diagnose, and fight illness. Immunologic medicine focuses on the dysfunctions of the immune system itself.

Immunodeficiency occurs when one or more of the body's protective elements is missing, scarce, or not working properly. Recurrent symptoms are one of the most common signs of such conditions.

A deficiency may involve just one aspect of a single immune system component's ability to function. For instance, to destroy an arthritis-causing intruder such as a bacterium, macrophages must be able to migrate to the site of an infection, adhere to the wall of a nearby blood vessel, ingest the foreign pain-causing substance, and activate powerful enzymes.

In arthritic conditions, the "big eater" cells are able to accomplish each of these steps if they are properly nourished with required nutrients. Niacinamide is needed to conduct the biochemical activities required for casting out arthritis-causing infections.

If there is a deficiency in niacinamide, for example, there is a defect in the delicately balanced complement chain and the chemicals called inhibitors that regulate its components.

Immune-deficiency conditions can be corrected when adequate nutrition is supplied to help correct the defect and strengthen the fortress against foreign invaders.

"A NIACINAMIDE A DAY KEEPS ARTHRITIS AWAY"

Many arthritics have been able to strengthen the immune system by taking a 25 milligram tablet of niacinamide every day. (Health stores and nutrition centers have this vitamin available. No prescription is required but your deficiency should be verified by a health practitioner.) For severe cases, a 300 milligram tablet is reported to be extremely beneficial in boosting the immune system and sending forth a full-fledged defensive attack against these invaders.

One former arthritic who was diagnosed as having a nutritional deficiency managed to recover rapidly by taking a 100 milligram tablet of niacinamide daily. She boasted that "A niacinamide a day keeps arthritis away!" Many others are able to experience freedom from joint stiffness through a correction in the immune defect system.

TWO IMMUNE-BOOSTING "ANTI-ARTHRITIS" FOODS THAT PROMOTE SWIFT HEALING

A powerhouse of niacinamide as well as most of the other B-complex vitamins will be found in two foods available at most health stores and supermarkets:

Brewer's Yeast—an almost "perfect" food with valuable niacinamide and minerals and protein needed to invigorate the sluggish immune system; it helps uproot and cast out the infectious substances that are to blame for joint stiffness.

Desiccated Liver—a food made out of liver but with the fat and connective tissue removed. It is rich in niacinamide together with the B-complex vitamins and unique amino acids with minerals; they counterattack bacterial invaders responsible for arthritic stiffness and pain.

To boost the power of your immune system, you may include these two foods in several swift-working, easily prepared beverages:

"Feel Good Yeast Brew"

In a glass of vegetable juice, stir in 1 teaspoon of brewer's yeast. Stir vigorously. Add a squeeze of lemon juice for Vitamin C. You could add a pinch of onion flakes for more piquant flavor. Drink at noontime when your body metabolism is at a higher level than the morning. One "Feel Good Yeast Brew" each day will supply niacinamide to your immune system and help promote joint flexibility very swiftly.

"Vitality Liver Drink"

Add 1 tablespoon of desiccated liver granules to one glass of tomato juice. Squeeze in the juice of one-half lemon or lime. Sprinkle with mixed herbs for a delicate flavor. Drink about one hour before your main or dinner meal when your metabolic processes are working at full speed. The "Vitality Liver Drink" will wake up a sluggish immune system, helping to eliminate irritants and infectious invaders so you will have more freedom from arthritic stiffness.

HOW THESE FOODS CORRECT IMMUNE DEFICIENCY AND IMPROVE JOINT FLEXIBILITY

The two preceding beverages are rich concentrates of niacinamide which is needed to alert the formation of pain-killing prostaglandins which also help cool off inflammation.

The combination of unique B-complex vitamins, minerals, and amino acids boosts a speedy reaction to your immune system. Within moments, the T-lymphocyte cells use the phagocytes to help uproot and cast out hurtful bacteria. The nutrients in these beverages use messenger proteins known as *lymphokines* to ease pain and stiffness. These lymphokines also stimulate production of interferon, a valuable immune response needed to ease and overcome arthritic pain.

The beverages use nutrients to assist helper T-cells, and suppressor T-cells curb the action of infectious bacteria. The nutrients enable protective cells to recognize a particle as an enemy. The cells then release antibodies which patrol the bloodstream, zero in on the invaders, hook precisely into them, and assist in casting them out of your body.

The rich concentration of nutrients with niacinamide at the forefront is the key to freedom from joint stiffness with these two foods. Niacinamide may work singly, but for many the related B vitamins are required for a strong and anti-arthritis immune system healing.

A MONTH OF NIACINAMIDE ENDS
YEARS OF ARTHRITIS

At age 58, Bertha U. had so much difficulty in reaching high shelves or bending over at waist level, she neglected household activities. Her movements were painfully restricted. Arthritis had "twisted" her hands and soon spread to her knees and ankles. All she could face now was a wheelchair, or possibly a walker that made her feel like an invalid.

Her neurologist decided to try nutritional therapy when new tests confirmed she had a niacinamide deficiency as well as below-normal levels of other B-complex vitamins. She was told to take either the "Feel Good Yeast Brew" or "Vitality Liver Drink" every single day. Because drugs made her feel sick, she was willing (although skeptical) to try nutritional remedies.

Within ten days on the niacinamide program, she felt her arms and hips becoming less painful and more agile. By the third week, she could use her hands, hips, knees, and ankles as if arthritis never struck. By the fourth week, Bertha U. was so agile, she could play a round of golf, do gardening, drive her car for hours (formerly unable because of arthritic stiffness), and enjoy square dancing until the wee hours of the night when others were exhausted! The walker was donated to a needy person with the advice that niacinamide could be a better solution if given a chance!

A BALANCE OF B-COMPLEX RESTORES
TOTAL DEFENSE

The condition of immunodeficiency is likely to happen when one or more of the body's protective forces is missing or not working properly. In some situations, arthritis linked to a deficiency of needed antibodies can be corrected with the use of niacinamide. In many others, the related "family" of B-complex vitamins are required to help fill the gap and "plug the hole" that has admitted foreign organisms.

A clinical examination will reveal nutritional deficiencies and the need for niacinamide and/or other nutrients for a strong immune system—the first line of defense against arthritis.

IN REVIEW

1. Vitamin B3 or niacinamide stimulates the immune system to release protective T-cells that help rid the body of irritants responsible for arthritic symptoms.

2. Joint stiffness and unsteady feet along with the risk of falling may be corrected with niacinamide.

3. Plan your menu to include the variety of tasty niacinamide-containing foods in daily meals. Feed yourself immunity to arthritis!

4. Anna E. became youthfully flexible in one day with the Morning Arthritis Tonic. It supercharged her immune system with bacteria-fighting macrophages and cast out arthritis.

5. A supervised supplement program may include niacinamide tablets to work swiftly in repairing a defect in the immune system.

6. Include either or both of the "anti-arthritis" foods that revitalize your immune system rapidly.

7. Either the "Feel Good Yeast Brew" or "Vitality Liver Drink" will give you the full spectrum of the entire B-complex group of vitamins along with other essential immune-nourishing nutrients.

8. Bertha U. ended years of arthritis within 30 days of niacinamide intake. Simple. Swift. Successful!

5

How to Use Vitamins as Pain Erasers

One of the most obvious signs of a deficiency in the immune system is the discomfort and pain of arthritis. If certain nutrients are either missing or in poor supply, the immune system weakens so that it is difficult to ward off the bacterial invasion responsible for arthritic distress. Pain, inflammatory or not, accompanied by swelling or with few visible appearances, is a warning symptom of a malnourished immune system.

Drugs Have Limitations and Risks

An assortment of antibiotics and antiviral drugs are said to help boost the diminished power of the immune system. Yet they are not able to cure its deficiencies. Medications act as reinforcements in the immunological system, but these chemical aids will not help the body's immune system build up additional potential immunity against future arthritic pain attacks.

Moreover, only so much additional strength can be introduced into the immune system. If the nutritional reserves are already too low, little can be done as the infectious invaders continue to take over. Drugs do have their side effects which many learn could be even worse than the condition itself. A natural alternative would seem to be the answer to the problem of arthritic pain. Vitamins have been found to effectively ease and erase pain and often help make arthritis "go away."

VITAMINS CREATE IMMUNITY TO PAIN

Vitamins are able to alert the immune system to create macrophages. These are uniquely special cells that play a vital role in fighting off immune system invaders that threaten the body with pain. Vitamins are needed to stimulate the immune system and activate the release of these immunostimulating macrophages. Vitamins have been found to be crucial pain erasing components in the immune system.

VITAMIN B6 (PYRIDOXINE)—ARTHRITIS FIGHTER

Scientists recognize that Vitamin B6 helps keep the body's immune system healthy in many ways. Animal studies have shown that white blood cells need B6 to produce antibodies. And the thymus gland, an important part of the immune system, needs B6 to command its legions of lymphocytes known as T-cells.

T-cells are one of the body's major defenses against invading enemies. They seek out, lock onto, and destroy these harmful substances. But they need B6 to do their job.

Scientific Discovery

Researchers at Oregon State University, Corvallis discovered that the T-cells of B6-deficient animals just did not have the energy to fight off a virus-induced invasion. "Getting enough B6 was important for T-cell activity, and enhanced the animals' ability to resist invasion," says a researcher.[1]

THE DOCTOR WHO HEALS PAINFUL HANDS

John M. Ellis, M.D., a family doctor from Mt. Pleasant, Texas, first discovered the value of Vitamin B6 as an immune stimulant to ease painful hands. In his highly acclaimed book,

---

[1] *Prevention Magazine,* April, 1985.

Dr. Ellis describes his experience in treating thousands of arthritic patients with Vitamin B6 or pyridoxine.

Pain, Swelling Is Eased

Dr. Ellis noted a pattern to the symptoms that would respond to an immune system strengthened by Vitamin B6; namely, swelling, numbness, tingling, reduced sense of touch in the fingers and hands, and pain in the finger joints, which impaired hand movements and weakened the grip.

Vitamin Invigorates Immune System

Dr. Ellis reports the vitamin stimulated the immune system to further heal even more "severe" cases. Patients suffered pain and stiffness in the shoulders and sometimes the elbows as well. Some had pain and/or swelling in the knees, the muscles between the shoulders and elbows, or the arms and chest. Some others had muscle spasms in the back of the legs and arches of the feet; most significant were locking of the finger joints and restless legs. It was Vitamin B6 that provided relief from these so-called "hopeless" symptoms.

Simple Daily Vitamin Program

The doctor would prescribe 50 milligrams a day of Vitamin B6 and noted that this entire group of symptoms would usually respond and go away, provided they had not been caused by an injury.

Relieve Tingling, Overweight, Nodes

"Aside from relieving the pain and swelling," Dr. Ellis says, "Vitamin B6 therapy helped arthritis patients whose arms would 'fall asleep' at night. Many would lose 5 to 7 pounds following B6 treatment, apparently because the vitamin helped eliminate excess fluid.

"In some cases, Heberden's nodes (small bony protrusions near the fingertips) shrank and became less painful." Dr. Ellis found Vitamin B6 to be most effective in middle-aged women with Heberden's nodes and arthritis of the interphalangeal joints (the middle group of knuckles), a symptom often diagnosed as "menopausal arthritis."

Immune System Provides Quick Relief

The B6-invigorated immune system worked swiftly. Relief frequently was felt after several days and progressed as the B6 treatment continued. The vitamin helped the immune system cast out invaders and thereby relieve elbow pain and improved finger flexion in about six weeks. "Nocturnal arm paralysis, muscle cramps, weak grip, and tactile sensation usually improved within two weeks," says Dr. Ellis.[2]

NUTRITIONAL THERAPY HEALS PAINFUL SYMPTOMS

Helen Y. was troubled with musculoskeletal symptoms and "chronic soreness" in her arms, neck, and shoulder. Medications produced intolerable abdominal pain. Her osteopathic physician conducted tests to learn she was deficient in Vitamin B6. He prescribed Vitamin B6, 50 milligrams a day, with another B-complex tablet containing 25 milligrams of each of the B-complex vitamins. For general immune boosting, she also took a multiple vitamin and mineral tablet. After three weeks, the painful swelling subsided and she became considerably better. The soreness was almost entirely gone by the end of the fourth week. Her immune system had "buffered" her pain and shielded her from hurtful invaders. All this because of nutritional healing.

A DOCTOR'S PLAN TO END ARTHRITIC PAIN

Arnold Fox, M.D., noted California internist and cardiologist, has found that certain vitamins and other nutrients are able to help stimulate the immune system and end chronic pain associated with arthritis. Below is his basic program.

ACE AGAINST ARTHRITIS

ACE forms the base of the anti-arthritis supplementation program I put most of my arthritis patients on. ACE stands for Vitamins A, C, and E. Individual needs vary and I cannot

---

[2] John M. Ellis, M.D., *Vitamin B6: The Doctor's Report,* Harper & Row, 1973, pp. 39–73.

prescribe vitamins and minerals without first examining a patient. But here is the general regimen I put most of my arthritic patients on:

VITAMIN A—10,000 IU of Vitamin A, *plus* plenty of beta-carotene from vegetables and fruits. For beta-carotene, eat two or three carrots a day, plus green and orange vegetables and orange fruits often.

B VITAMINS—I suggest to my patients a B-complex vitamin containing 60 milligrams of the major B vitamins. I have them take 1 tablet, twice a day. In addition to the B-complex, I recommend boosters of the following members:

NIACIN—25 milligrams, three times a day. Gradually increase the dose to 100 milligrams three times a day. If an unpleasant flush develops on the face or body, reduce the dosage until the flush disappears. Niacin seems to decrease joint stiffness and the deformity associated with arthritis.

NIACINAMIDE—for the very severe cases of arthritis, 500 milligrams three times a day. Niacinamide is also a form of niacin but does not cause a flush.

VITAMIN B6—500 milligrams twice a day, once after breakfast and once after lunch. During an arthritis flareup, the dosage is doubled to two 500 milligram tablets after breakfast and two 500 milligram tablets after lunch.

VITAMIN C—As with Vitamin A, I have my patients taking two kinds of Vitamin C. First is a buffered Vitamin C powder, a hypoallergenic formula that contains the following in 1 teaspoon: 2,350 milligrams Vitamin C; 450 milligrams Calcium, 250 milligrams of magnesium, and 99 milligrams of potassium.

Benefit: With this buffered form of Vitamin C (pH 6.3), the side effects sometimes seen with regular Vitamin C are avoided. I have my patients take 1 teaspoon in a glass of water or juice with breakfast.

In Addition: I have my arthritic patients take 1,000 milligrams of Vitamin C in tablet form, three times a day, with meals. If they are enjoying at least a 50 percent improvement and feeling good at the end of four weeks, I have them stick with this dosage. If not, I usually have them take 2,000 milligrams three times a day, with meals.

VITAMIN E—400 milligrams of D-alpha tocopherol (Vitamin E) twice a day, once after breakfast and once after lunch. I prefer the water-soluble form, available as a dry powder in a soft gelatin capsule. Vitamin E is an antioxidant which some authorities suggest slows the rate of aging and does seem to slow the formation of arthritis.

MINERALS—I have my patients begin with a multiple mineral that contains one-quarter of the recommended daily allowance (RDA) for all the minerals, and take four tablets a day. In addition to the multiple mineral, I suggest to my patients:

SELENIUM—200 micrograms a day. Selenium is a potent free radical quencher and an anti-aging ally of Vitamin E.

ZINC—220 milligrams of zinc sulfate (50 milligrams of elemental zinc) a day, but twice a day during an arthritis flareup.

Dr. Fox comments, "I vary this plan according to an individual's needs, giving more or less as is indicated."[3]

PAIN-FREE IN FOUR DAYS

Edith Q. endured arthritis for many years. It began in her knees and gradually spread to her shoulders and hands. She injured herself when she fell down on her left elbow and that worsened her arthritis. She tried aspirins but complained they made her sick.

When treated by an internist, tests showed she had difficulties with her weakened immune system. To stimulate the production of macrophages and bacteria-fighting T-lymphocytes, Edith Q. was put on the aforedescribed nutritional program.

Almost from the start, she began to feel better. Within four days, she had almost no pain. Swelling had gone down. She could walk for blocks and blocks without any wringing spasms of pain that restricted movements. Her immune system was sufficiently invigorated to cast out hurtful infections and build

---

[3] Arnold Fox, M.D., *DLPA to End Chronic Pain and Depression,* Pocket Books, 1985, pp. 112–114.

a strong resistance to painful arthritis. Nutrition had promoted healing.

VITAMINS REVITALIZE IMMUNE SYSTEM

The importance of vitamins is underscored by noted arthritis specialist, Robert Bingham, M.D., of Desert Hot Springs, California, who zeroes in on these specific groups:

Vitamins B and C are below normal in most arthritis patients and invariably low in cases of rheumatoid arthritis. Chronic low intake of these vitamins predisposes to lowered resistance against disease, particularly those of virus origin which long have been suspected as the cause of rheumatoid arthritis. These vitamins are water-soluble and not stored in the body so they must be obtained from fresh fruits, vegetables, nuts, and whole grains. Depletion of the B-complex and C vitamins occurs in stress and exhaustion, after surgical operations, illnesses, and injuries. A deficiency of only a short time can make a patient's joints more susceptible to the onset of acute arthritis.

Vitamin D is most important. Most patients on the so-called average American diet receive only about 5 percent of their normal daily requirement of Vitamin D. Since it is essential for bone metabolism and has been found to act as a steroid hormone, any Vitamin D deficiency results in joint damage and lack of bone replacement and repair.

Dr. Bingham comments, "Unexpected deficiencies which produce a sort of 'metabolic poor health' do not necessarily cause arthritis but certainly decrease the chances of recovery. In order to adequately determine a patient's nutritional deficiencies and take steps to correct them, laboratory analysis is essential. The type and degree of nutritional deficiency can be determined by means of a detailed dietary diagnosis."[4]

NUTRITIONAL THERAPY BOOSTS IMMUNE BARRIER

In a healthy immune system, the lymphocytes (T-cells and B-cells) perform the crucial task of recognizing foreign or unhealthy invaders. They do so by means of receptors or protein

---

[4] Robert Bingham, M.D., Desert Hot Springs, California, personal communication.

molecules on their surfaces. This process calls for adequate nutrition so that the lymphocyte receptors are able to distinguish possible causes of harm from the body's own normal constituents, and to use exactly the right tactics and weapons against each one. To initiate this arthritis-fighting process, nutrition does play a key if not a decisive role.

Dr. Robert Bingham explains, "Diseases of the bones and joints which are due to deficiencies in a single nutritional factor are many. They include scurvy, a Vitamin C deficiency; osteoporosis, from lack of calcium and protein; neuropathy, from Vitamin B-complex deficiency; and degenerative joint disease due to a combination of nutritional deficiencies.

Furthermore, Dr. Bingham says these same nutritional deficiencies open the door to many of the infectious diseases by lowering the natural resistance of the body to bacteria, viruses, and parasites.

This further emphasizes the relationship between nutrition and arthritis, because "secondary arthritis is often caused by diseases which interfere with the absorption, digestion, and metabolism of certain vital nutritional factors." Such conditions include disturbances of the digestive system, food allergies, endocrine (glandular) diseases, and the changes in body chemistry associated with menopause and the aging processes of the body.

IMMUNE SYSTEM WEAKNESS NEEDS
TO BE DETECTED

Dr. Bingham notes that while advanced nutritional deficiencies can be recognized by the medical practitioner, "subclinical deficiencies, usually too small to be detected by ordinary means, usually multiple in their existence and occurring over a period of years, may bring on more subtle changes in the bones and joints and result in degenerative bone and joint disease. This used to be considered a disease of old age, but in our era of 'civilized foods' with its increased use of nutritionally poor foodstuffs, we are seeing this condition in more and more young people. We are not surprised to find it in the 30s and 40s, where our medical authorities taught us to expect it in the 60s and 70s."

Dr. Bingham feels that many arthritics can be helped via strengthening the immune system as early as possible with nutritional therapy.

IMPORTANT ROLE FOR VITAMIN C IN IMMUNE REBUILDING

Vitamin C has long been recognized as important in rebuilding and strengthening a weak immune system to help correct arthritis and ease the pain involved.

Vitamin C Benefits

This vitamin helps thin the synovial fluid (lubricating fluid of the joints), allowing easier movement and less incidence of pain. It stimulates the immune system to maintain blood vessel integrity. It is also involved in the normal formation of collagen (a substance important in building connective tissue); it is an important factor in strengthening the immune system to resist invasion of hurtful substances.

For many arthritics, Vitamin C is needed to rebuild the immune barrier to provide a shield against bacteria, viruses, and other pain-causing microorganisms.

HOW TO EAT AND DRINK YOUR WAY TO PAIN RELIEF

Include this pain-relieving nutrient in your meal program throughout the day and give your immune system a boost to help the lymphocyte cells uproot and cast out painful bacteria. Some tasty ways to eat your way to freedom from arthritic pain include the following:

Morning Relaxant. In a glass of skim milk, stir in 1 teaspoon of ascorbic acid powder. Stir vigorously and drink slowly.

Vitamin C Salad. Arrange freshly washed turnip greens, red and green peppers, broccoli, and kale on a bed of greens. Sprinkle with ascorbic acid powder. Top with several strawberries.

Fruits to Ease Distress. On seasonal greens, spread straw-berries, guava slices, papaya slices, orange and tangerine wedges. Sprinkle with ascorbic acid powder. A powerhouse of Vitamin C and minerals that help relax the throbbing pain.

Berry Juice. Blenderize an assortment of high Vitamin C berries such as strawberries, gooseberries, raspberries, and black-berries. Drink whenever you feel pain coming on.

Vegetable Tonic. Blenderize or juice cabbage, red and green peppers, tomatoes, turnip greens, kale, broccoli, and Brussels sprouts. Add a bit of lemon juice for a spicy flavor. (You need not use all vegetables at the same time but an assortment of what is seasonally available.) Drink one or two glasses daily.

Bedtime Beverage. A glass of cabbage juice is a strong supply of Vitamin C. A squeeze of lemon or lime juice gives a tasty flavor. Taken at bedtime, it induces comfort and con-tentment and ease of pain so you can sleep with a minimum of arthritis upset.

Arthritis-Soothing Elixir. In a glass of grapefruit juice, stir in 1 teaspoon of ascorbic acid powder. Break a niacinamide tablet and mix into the elixir. You have a unique combination of vitamins that utilize the power of the phagocytes, neutrophils, and macrophages which are taken up by the lymphocytes to rid the body of pain-causing substances.

You can strike back at arthritis pain with the use of Vitamin C as a first line of defense against hurtful bacteria.

DRINKS HIS WAY TO FREEDOM FROM ARTHRITIS PAIN

Working on a computer was easy for Morton J. B. until he began to experience severe wrist, knuckle, and shoulder pains. He had such twisting pain, he slowed up in his work to the point where he could have faced dismissal. His fingers were not as flexible as required for the computer terminal and word processing machines he had used for years and years.

Aspirins and medications made Morton J. B. groggy so much that he misinterpreted verbal instructions and garbled up his work. He faced job loss as well as career loss if he could not "get it together" as was suggested.

He heard a lecturing virologist and immunologist talk about the value of nutrition in rebuilding the immune system to "knock out" pain. He decided to give it a try. Morton J. B. brought a thermos to his computer terminal base and throughout the day would sip either a *Vegetable Tonic* or *Arthritis-Soothing Elixir* or *Morning Relaxant.* He alternated to give his body different tastes and combinations. Within four days, his knuckles and wrists became flexible as the pain was soothed. Within ten days, the pain was only a slight occasional tremor. He was able to think clearly because he eliminated aspirins and other upsetting drugs. His job was not only secure but since he was pain-free he worked so well he was soon slated for a promotion.

The potent nutrients had strengthened his immune system to cast out hurtful invaders. Morton J. B. was saved from arthritic pain and the threat of lifetime disability.

Give your immune system the needed nutrients to resist the invasion of painful outsiders. With vitamins and other nutrients, you will stimulate your immune system to help your body erase pain!

IN REVIEW

1. Vitamin B6 (pyridoxine) is recognized as an arthritis fighter and pain reliever.
2. A leading physician boosts the immune system and erases pain with the use of a single vitamin. It works quickly.
3. Helen Y. relieved musculoskeletal pain with the use of an easy vitamin formula that boosted immune system efficiency.
4. A leading California internist has found that a team of vitamins in specified amounts help ease pain and arthritis flareup.
5. Vitamin C is identified as a star in the hope for freedom from arthritis pain.
6. Edith Q. followed a simple vitamin program and experienced recovery from arthritis pain in four days.
7. Boost nutritional therapy with foods and beverages as described. Tasty and effective.
8. Morton J. B. used simply prepared beverages to drink away his arthritis pain which threatened his job and lifestyle.

6

How Nutritional Immunity Relieves Virus-Caused Arthritis Pain . . . in Minutes

The invader is tiny, about one sixteen-thousandth the size of the head of a pin. It is a virus, or chemical particle, that is smaller than a bacterium. Visible only with an electron microscope, most viruses consist of an outer shell or *capsid* that in some cases resembles a geodesic dome built of individual protein molecules. This shell protects the key ingredient, a molecule of genetic material (nucleic acid). When a virus invades a cell, the viral genes—which range in number from half a dozen to several hundred—supply the host cell with a "core" to make multiple copies of that particular virus.

Arthritis Virus Invades Body

Suppose an arthritis *virion*—a free viral particle consisting of a capsid and nucleic acid—chances upon a susceptible cell. How does it penetrate? A backup force prompts the arthritis virus to penetrate, disrupt the host cell's normal genetic and metabolic machinery, and bring about a defect in the immune system to create arthritic symptoms.

New virions are released from the cell by a process called *budding* in which the virion pushes out the cell membrane to form a bubble. This portion of membrane then pinches off, allowing the encapsulated virion to float free of the cell. Budding releases thousands of arthritis viral particles throughout the system. The newer knowledge of nutritional immunity recognizes a weakness that has allowed the enemy to invade and arthritis to strike.

THE IMMUNE SYSTEM TO THE RESCUE

As soon as the arthritis virus enters the body, the internal defense system moves into gear. When the invasion begins, the first defenders to scramble into the battle are the *macrophages*. These are large, white blood cells with protective instincts. They destroy invading viruses by engulfing and ingesting them. Debris, invaders, and damaged body cells are all swallowed up by the voracious macrophages.

Immune Powers Increase

With the use of nutrition, macrophages also help produce *interferon*—a group of small proteins that are a key component of viral immunity. Interferon is secreted not only by macrophages, but by other infected cells as well. Interferon cannot save damaged cells, but once released into the bloodstream, interferon bolsters healthy cells' ability to resist arthritis viral infection. A bonus is that nutritionally boosted interferon production in response to the invasion of one kind of virus also helps temporarily to block infection by other kinds.

Power of T-Cells

An important type of arthritis-fighting white blood cell, the T-cell, may be used for the immune reaction by macrophages. Different kinds of T-cells have different functions in arthritis-fighting. Some, referred to as "helper T-cells," are equipped for reconnaissance, marking viruses for destruction by latching onto structures called *antigens* found on the surfaces of macrophages that have engulfed the viruses and emitting chemical signals that alert the rest of the system to the arthritis invader.

Other T-cells are known as "killer T-cells," even though they do not actually attack the virus particles. Killer T-cells are programmed to directly attack and kill infected cells. Interferon also helps activate killer T-cells.

Dynamic B-Cells

These are additional disease-fighting white blood cells that are called into the fray by helper T-cells. B-cells differentiate into specialized cells called *plasma cells* that secrete *antibody* molecules into the blood. The antibodies fit "lock-and-key" fashion into the invading viruses' antigens. This binding renders the viruses harmless and labels them for elimination. Antibodies also bind to virus-infected cells and attract macrophages and T-cells to destroy the infected cells. Viruses, however, often spread so quickly from cell to cell that they elude the antibodies.

Complement System

Macrophages respond to the complement system—blood proteins activated in a series of stages like an internal fountain of youth. These destroy arthritic invaders either by punching fatal holes in them or by marking them to attract killer T-cells or macrophages.

Nutrition Creates Immune Power

Nutrients are needed to utilize all of these factors in the vital *lymphokine* production—the provision of B-cell growth factor, interleukin, and other arthritis-fighting immune responses. One weak nutritional link in this chain and the arthritis virus is able to suppress the body's defenses and, in fact, suppress your immune system. The pain and debilitation of arthritis then takes root.

HOW NUTRITION SHIELDS AGAINST ARTHRITIS INFECTION

Immunologists have discovered a possible cause of arthritis. The surface of an invading virus becomes infected with a substance called *human leukocyte antigen* or HLA. This molecule is believed linked to a breakdown in the immune system. Nutritional scientists believe that T-cells have the ability to recognize the arthritic pain-causing HLA molecule and create a form of inner immunity.

T-cells are responsible for turning on the immune system in all of its forms. The various immune defenses include production of antibodies to attack the arthritic invader, to stimulate other T-cells to attack cells infected by arthritis.

Scientists have noted that in order for the T-cells to set off the shielding immune system, they must first be activated by another cell. Namely, the macrophages or scavenger cells are empowered to form antibodies. The macrophages ingest the arthritis virus. They weaken the HLA molecules. Then T-cells are alerted, carried by the bloodstream. The T-cells "see" the arthritis viral fragments presented to them by the macrophages, and—in a counter-attack against the invader—activate the immune system to attack the invader—activate the immune system to attack that particular arthritis virus wherever it is found.

This process requires important nutrients for vigor and power. If the body is weak or deficient in nutrients, then the process becomes correspondingly weak. The arthritic develops an autoimmune condition in which the T-cells do not recognize the infectious virus and the condition spreads. Some T-cells attack the body's own defenses and trigger antibodies against these important defenses to create weakness. The body loses its ability to shield itself against arthritis among other conditions.

THE VITAMIN THAT FIGHTS VIRUS ENEMIES

Vitamin C helps to inhibit virus intrusion into the cells. It is essential in the formation of macrophages, the white blood cells or the immune system's "hit men." Your immune system uses Vitamin C to manufacture the T- and B-cells and also the powerful antibodies that can identify the arthritis virus and defuse its threat to your health.

Vitamin C Is a Virus-Buster

Vitamin C is a powerful detoxifier of the arthritis virus. It neutralizes most toxic wastes, both those produced in the body and those picked up from the environment. It stimulates the production of arthritis-fighting antibodies and white blood cells and inhibits the growth of risky pathogenic viruses or bacteria.

How to Boost the Immune System with a Virus-Buster Vitamin

Boost consumption of citrus fruits and juices on a daily basis. Use grapefruits, oranges, and tangerines as a dessert, as a snack, as part of a daily salad with seasonal greens. Drink their juices as a thirst-quencher. You will be boosting your body's immune response with Vitamin C needed to initiate T- and B-cell production to fight arthritis virus infection.

Virus-Buster Punch

In a glass of citrus juice, stir in 1 teaspoon of Vitamin C powder and 1 teaspoon of rose hips powder (from a health store). Stir vigorously. Drink in the early afternoon when your metabolic processes are more active. Within moments, the rich concentrate of Vitamin C will nourish your glands and stimulate your immune system to give power to the T- and B-cells, to produce interferon and to help "bust" viral infections. The rose hips is a "punch" that knocks out arthritis virus threats. Rose hips is made from the fruit of the blooming rose and is one of the most powerful concentrated sources of the virus buster.

VIRUS-BUSTER PUNCH KNOCKS OUT ARTHRITIS IN DAYS

Jean G. needed to be in top shape to meet daily responsibilities. They called for managing a special department in the school system, maintaining a home for her husband and three active children, and also participating in many local social functions.

Wear and tear had never been a problem until she began to feel a stiff shoulder. Before long, Jean G. would grimace with pain when getting up from her seat. Driving to and fro became a hurtful experience. Morning stiffness slowed her up. She was frequently late for meetings. Schedules started to slip. She was hardly a good example of punctuality to students and family. Would she be restricted with the onset of arthritis? Her wrists were so stiff, she could scarcely write on a blackboard or do housework. Medications offered some relief but made her sleepy and unable to speak clearly. She could feel her world collapsing.

A laboratory technician who specializes in viral infections urged her to obtain diagnostic tests to see if her arthritis was traced to a nutritional weakness in her immune system. It was! A report indicated she needed a nutritional support treatment with emphasis upon Vitamin C.

Jean G. started consumption of citrus fruits and juices and the "powerhouse" special—the Virus-Buster Punch. Within ten days, her shoulders and wrists were flexible. She awoke with agile joints, could move about easily. Within 20 days, the nutritional vigor had strengthened her immune system to cast out the hurtful virus. She was alert and active. Her school system position, household, and social life were back on a happy and vigorous schedule. Her immune system had responded to nutritional therapy to seek and destroy the arthritis virus.

VITAMIN A—AMAZING "CLEANSER" OF ARTHRITIS VIRUS

Can you cleanse your system of any virus that is believed responsible for arthritis? The answer is that one special vitamin is spotlighted as being able to muster your immune system and sweep out potentially harmful and hurtful arthritis virus invaders.

Vitamin A and Immune-Boosting Cell Oxygenation

Vitamin A or its vegetable source, beta-carotene, increases the permeability of blood capillaries. These capillaries carry oxygen and other nutritive substances to your T-cells and B-cells to enable them to alert the virus-fighting and immune-protecting macrophages.

The more permeable the capillary walls, the more oxygen can be delivered to your virus-fighting cells. It is Vitamin A that boosts cell oxygenation; or, it gives the "breath of life" to the cells, to cause the complement system to distribute needed antibodies to "knock out" the arthritis virus.

Vitamin A cleanses the destroyed virus fragments from your body. At the same time, it boosts immunity by regulating the strength and tensile stability of tissues in your cell walls. This protects against a breakdown of cell membranes; if this happens, foreign invaders enter and have "free play" in your body and are involved in a breakdown in the immune system. It is Vitamin A that helps protect against these gaps.

Food Sources of Vitamin A

These are found in two groups, meat as well as meatless:

Meat Group: Liver, whole egg, cheddar cheese, as well as milk products (read label for potency). You may be concerned about the cholesterol and fat content of these sources and want to keep them to a minimum. Or else, try an alternative source.

Meatless Group: Sweet potato, corn on the cob, cooked carrots, squash, broccoli, asparagus, cantaloupe, mango, apricots, peaches, nectarines. These foods have no cholesterol and offer Vitamin A in the form of beta-carotene which is then transformed into a usable vitamin by your body. Some sources of beta-carotene will be found in green, leafy vegetables although their color is masked by the green pigment chlorophyll.

Easy Way to Feed Vitamin A to Your Immune System

Include a variety of the preceding meatless foods in your daily menu. Also enjoy fresh raw juices made from these vegetables and fruits for potent beta-carotene. Meat foods may also be included although in modest amounts if you are cautious about excess cholesterol and fat.

CORRECTS IMMUNE SYSTEM DEFICIENCY WITH BETA-CAROTENE

"What, me have arthritis? How is that possible?" Susan M. was shaken when her homeopathic physician diagnosed her shooting spasms and painful "knots" in her lower back. Her knees were so stiff she could barely commute to her systems analyst position in the next town. Her reflexes were slowed because of increasing pain as well as recurring inflammation.

Her homeopathic physician explained that a nutritional deficiency had weakened her immune system. Repeated attacks of arthritis virus invaders had overcome the barriers so that her T- and B-cells were unable to cope with the corrosive threat.

Susan M. was told to increase Vitamin C and balanced minerals but the diagnosis indicated she needed boosting of beta-carotene. She included the assortment of foods with this immune-feeding nutrient. In her particular situation, she had a marked deficiency of Vitamin A and needed extra fortification to strengthen the immune barrier.

Fresh fruits and vegetables as well as their juices worked wonders within three weeks. Her pains and "knots" were "melted" and she could move with agility. Reflexes were alert again and inflammation was all but entirely cooled.

The beta-carotene nourished her T- and B-cells to send forth virus cleansing macrophages so that the arthritis invaders could be "cleansed" from her system. She calls beta-carotene her "natural arthritis medicine."

VITAMIN E HELPS BUILD ARTHRITIS IMMUNITY

Viruses are believed to be the single most common cause of illness and many have traced a close connection between viruses and the immune system. To build resistance to arthritis and to help eliminate the infection, nutrition is one of the most potent forces.

Every moment of your life, your body creates 200,000 new immune cells and thousands of antibody molecules. To create this protection, your body needs the right supply of vitamins, minerals, proteins, and other elements. In particular, immunologists have found that Vitamin E is essential in helping to build arthritis resistance as well as eventual healing.

Stress, Body Aging, Free Radicals

Stress weakens the body's defenses to pave the way to viral invasion. During normal aging, the oxygenation of your cells is diminished. Because of increased rancidity of fats, certain substances called free radicals are formed within the cells. These free radicals have a destructive effect on normal cell metabolism, causing a weakening of the T-cells and B-cells and a reduction in macrophage production. Arthritis can take root as virus invaders are able to spread without the counter-attack of antibodies. In many situations, boosting Vitamin E can help forestall and reverse this threat to your immune system.

Vitamin E Strengthens Immune Responses

This virus-busting vitamin increases the body's resistance to stress by improving circulation, preventing harmful oxidation of fats, and increasing the supply of oxygen to the cells and tissues. Vitamin E is an antioxidant at the cellular level; since one of the understandings of arthritis is that there is an accumulation of free radicals resulting from oxidative reactions in the body, the use of Vitamin E as an immune-strengthening nutrient is to be considered.

Vitamin E helps the immune system produce an antibody that recognizes and goes after a particular antigen or invader. Helper T-cells and B-cells, and macrophages, are sent to destroy the arthritis invader.

Food Sources of Vitamin E

Whole grains, seeds, nuts, cold-pressed vegetable oils, wheat germ, green leafy vegetables.

Important: It is well to note that a high intake of polyunsaturated fatty acids, found in vegetable oils, increases your need for Vitamin E. Although oils are considered a good source of this vitamin, there could be losses occurring during the refining process. Careful storage of oils is important since rancidity causes Vitamin E losses. Heating oils to high temperature also reduces their Vitamin E content as well as the freezing of fried foods.

Vitamin E in capsule form is available in health stores, pharmacies, and many supermarkets. As part of a total nutritional immunity program, supplements may often be required.

KNOCKS OUT ARTHRITIS IN MINUTES WITH VITAMIN E

Department store supervisor, Tom W., also doubled as storeroom stacker during slack days. He had always been able to move cartons around with speed and agility, rarely requiring the help of the shipping room staff. But one afternoon, he felt a knife-like stab in his lumbar (lower) region while moving one small packing box to another location in the warehouse. It was the start of what was later diagnosed as arthritis.

His osteopathic physician conducted thorough laboratory tests and examinations to note that Tom W. had allowed himself to become deficient in beta-carotene but especially in Vitamin E. He hardly ever ate whole grains or used oils; he insisted he ate lots of bread in sandwiches and other forms but it was a refined, bleached, cottony product with the Vitamin E non-existent because of processing. His immune system was "starved" for this important virus-busting vitamin!

The problem was a weakness in his T- and B-cell production. Harmful arthritis virus invaders had taken root and were causing the insidious symptoms. As part of a nutritional boosting program, his osteopathic physician suggested supplements of Vitamin E together with the dietary change of enjoying whole grains whether in bread or cereals or in oils.

Within minutes after starting the program, Tom W. was relieved of low-back and body pain. Before the day ended, he could perform with the agility of a healthy person. He was able to knock out the arthritis virus in minutes with the unique Vitamin E program. Because of his physical energy, he was soon given a bonus and promotion. "I owe it all to my immune system," he says with a smile. "And to Vitamin E . . . for excellence!"

QUICK WAYS TO FEED VITAMIN E TO THE IMMUNE SYSTEM

Strengthen your immune system; cast out hurtful arthritis-causing free radicals; enjoy a soothing, pain-free contentment with Vitamin E in any of these tasty ways:

*Break open a Vitamin E capsule and sprinkle over any raw salad.

*Use seeds and nuts with raisins for a Vitamin E and Vitamin C powerhouse to infuse new strength into your T- and B-cells.

*Enjoy a green, leafy vegetable sprinkled with raw wheat germ and a bit of a cold-pressed vegetable oil. Diced seeds and nuts add piquant taste and more Vitamin E.

*Blenderize some wheat germ oil in any vegetable juice and enjoy as an immune-building beverage.

*Sprinkle raw wheat germ over any salad or add to any whole grain cereal with sun-dried raisins for a rich concentrate of Vitamin E among other nutrients.

*Use cold-pressed oils as part of a salad dressing when combined with some apple cider vinegar and honey. Energizing!

VITAMINS ARE ACTIVE VIRUS-BUSTERS

Your immune system requires a balanced nutritional plan to help screen out potentially hurtful and threatening arthritis invaders. In many situations, one vitamin may be more in need than the other. A thorough laboratory diagnosis as well as your own reactions will tell you how either one or more vitamins are needed to help "fight back" and cast out these hurtful arthritis invaders.

It is important to use nutritional therapy in boosting the immune system as early as possible. Some arthritis viruses "hide" in the body after their initial attack, only to emerge later in a much more virulent form. The ability of certain viruses to persist and replicate makes this deficiency possible. With the help of nutrition, your body is able to muster the process that will uproot and destroy this threat to your health. Nutrition can fight (and win) against the arthritis virus.

IN REVIEW

1. The probable cause of arthritis is believed to be a virus. With nutritional therapy, the immune system can be mustered to identify and evict this threat from your body.

2. Nutrition is able to mobilize the T- and B-cells to create immune cleansing and correction of the arthritis virus syndrome.

3. Vitamin C fights virus enemies. The Virus-Buster Punch is a powerhouse of corrective nutritional therapy. Works fast.

4. Jean G. used the Virus-Buster Punch to knock out her arthritis invasion in a matter of days.

5. Vitamin A is able to strengthen the walls of the immune system and wash out arthritis viral infections in a short time.

6. Susan M. used a vegetable form of Vitamin A to untie her painful arthritis knots and correct her immune system to resist this threat.

7. Vitamin E is a vital antioxidant that actually creates antibodies to destroy the arthritis virus.

8. Tom W.'s "backbreaking" arthritis was corrected with Vitamin E therapy. His regenerated immune system made him arthritis-free in days.

9. A balanced nutritional program helps strengthen the immune system and shield against arthritis, but you may need more of any (or all) of the important virus-fighting elements.

7

How Magic Minerals Rejuvenate Your Immune System to Cast Out Arthritis

Minerals may act as vaccines against viral infections that trigger arthritis infections. Because the turnover of minerals in the body is slower than that of vitamins, deficiencies take longer to develop. Yet they are keys to correction of defects in the immune system and can provide a knockout punch to an invading arthritis virus.

Minerals are important in the formation of the skeletal structure, the maintenance of your acid-base balance, and as catalysts (helpers) in biological reactions. They serve as regulators of muscle contractility, as transmitters of nerve impulses, and in the promotion of growth.

The newer knowledge of nutritional immunology has focused on the importance of minerals, whether in foods or supplements, in rejuvenating your immune system to help cast out arthritis.

ZINC ZAPS ARTHRITIS

Zinc is considered to be the most vital mineral for the immune system. Without enough zinc in your body, many of the lymph system tissues actually shrink, including the thymus where the crucial T-cells develop.

The concentration of zinc in your cells also affects how energetically protective antibodies attack arthritis invaders.

Zinc Power

Zinc musters the body's arthritis-fighting white blood cells to rout the invaders. Zinc ions come into direct contact with the hurtful viruses. It is believed that zinc inhibits the cleavage of viral polypeptides. The polypeptide cleavage takes place inside of a healthy cell that the virus has "hijacked," and cleavage must occur before a virus can clone itself. Zinc ions disrupt this process and correct against replication and "arthritis spread."

Zinc is also believed to work with Vitamin C to initiate the body's own production of interferon, a substance to protect against arthritis. Zinc plus Vitamin C initiate an outpouring of interferon which stops the arthritis virus from multiplying.

All cells have the ability to produce interferon but you can give that ability a shot in the arm by boosting your intake of both zinc and Vitamin C. In particular, zinc has been labeled as a natural virus killer because of its unique power.

Food Sources of Zinc

Whole grains, pumpkin seeds, and brewer's yeast are great sources. Wheat germ and wheat bran are rich concentrates. Other good sources are cowpeas (blackeye), skim milk, and brown rice.

SOOTHING SELENIUM FOR SWIFT ARTHRITIS RELIEF

Selenium is required for growth in human cells and helps protect against exudative diathesis (spontaneous swelling and hemorrhages). A unique relationship between selenium and arthritis invasion makes it clear that this mineral has the ability to fight off the threat of a harmful virus.

Selenium stimulates the immunological system in its work against the development of arthritis through its powerful antioxidant action. It reportedly helps prevent or slows down the formation of arthritic-like free radicals in the system. Selenium is a great protector and detoxifier and helps to minimize the effect of toxic chemicals which could cause virus infection.

Food Sources of Selenium

Brewer's yeast, garlic, liver, eggs, and brown rice are all fine sources. *Note:* Garlic is, singularly, gram for gram, the richest source of selenium. Garlic also contains a valuable immune-building mineral, germanium, which works with selenium to protect against cell invaders.

Even with plenty of characteristically selenium-rich foods, however, it is often difficult to obtain protective amounts of this mineral if foods were grown on selenium-poor soil.

One good form of supplementation would be brewer's yeast in moderate amounts. This immune-building mineral is also available in supplementary tablet form, and a general rule of thumb would be to take from 25 to 50 micrograms a day. *Caution:* Selenium is cumulative in the human body; therefore, supplements should be taken in small doses and under the guidance of your health practitioner.

CALCIUM FOR A STRONG ARTHRITIS-RESISTANT IMMUNE SYSTEM

The most abundant mineral in the body, most calcium is found in bones and teeth. A small amount present in blood plays a vital role in the regulation of muscle contraction and in the activation of several enzymes.

Your immune system depends upon calcium to establish equilibrium with phosphorus and magnesium and is closely related to a hormone secreted by the parathyroid glands. The efficient utilization of calcium depends on an adequate supply of Vitamin D.

Calcium is used by your immune system to strengthen your nervous and muscle networks and also to build and repair bone and cartilage.

A deficiency of calcium allows penetration of infectious agents that could trigger spontaneous cramping of the muscles and legs as well as the arthritic tenderness of muscles.

If your immune system is deficient in calcium, the infectious invaders create more arthritic difficulties. Soft bones at the edges of the joints become "irritated" and cannot tolerate pressures. Gradually "spurs" and "exostoses" are formed like little lips on the joint margins, a characteristic finding in the x-rays of many arthritic patients.

Food Source of Calcium

Hard cheeses, milk, leafy vegetables, beans, oranges, nuts, eggs, whole grains, chard, cauliflower, kale, dates, figs, almonds, walnuts, bran, oatmeal are good sources.

CALCIUM PROTECTS AGAINST POLLUTION

Arthritis infections may often be triggered when harmful fallout or pollution enters the body. It signals an erosion of the immune system and more hurtful invaders penetrate the barrier.

There have been links between lead poisoning and a breakdown in the immune system to pave the way to arthritis among other infections.

Lead comes into the atmosphere mostly from automobiles which burn gasoline treated with lead. It pollutes the air and enters your body to punch holes in your immune fortress. It is said that an average of over 200 million pounds of lead enter the atmosphere from automobile exhaust pipes each year— that's almost 1 pound per person!

Calcium is said to have a protective effect against lead and other toxic substances; for example, mercury and strontium 90, to which we are all subjected in this atomic age.

To help build resistance against pollution invaders, calcium is helpful as part of your nutritional program.

TASTY TIPS TO CALCIUM FORTIFICATION OF THE IMMUNE SYSTEM

There's more to calcium than drinking milk. You may want to select low-fat or non-fat milk as a primary source of calcium. Additional immune-boosting calcium tips include:

*Add low-salt and low-fat cheese to sandwiches.
*Snack on cheese and salt-free crackers.
*Prepare soups with milk instead of water.
*Add non-fat dry milk to soups, stews, and casseroles.
*Use milk and cheese in casseroles.
*Add grated cheese to Mexican and Italian foods such as tacos, lasagna, and ravioli.
*Add cheese to your salads.
*Eat yogurt with meals or as a snack.
*Make your desserts high in calcium—frozen yogurt, cheese with fruit, custards and puddings made with milk.
*Add non-fat dry milk to yogurt for a robust flavor and much more calcium.

Include Sunshine

Vitamin D which is produced in the skin by the sun's rays increases calcium absorption in your body. About 20 to 30 minutes of sunshine daily will help this process.

Exercise, Too

Calcium is better metabolized by your body to immunize against arthritis if you exercise regularly. About 30 minutes regularly will assist in this important immune-building function. Walking, doctor-approved jogging, swimming, or supervised health club activities are a few ways to exercise and keep immune.

CALCIUM ABSORPTION MADE SIMPLE

Absorption of calcium in the gastrointestinal system depends partly on the presence of hydrochloric acid in the stomach.

If you take excessive amounts of alkali or antacids for indigestion, or large amounts of buffered aspirin for pain, or if you have atrophy of the gastrointestinal lining, you may be deficient in hydrochloric acid.

The popular folk remedy of honey and apple cider vinegar for arthritis may be successful because it stimulates the formation of hydrochloric acid in the stomach; and the acid in the vinegar aids in calcium absorption.

Simple Technique: Mix 1 tablespoon of honey with 1 table-spoon of apple cider vinegar and sprinkle over a salad as you begin your meal. Or put the same combination in a glass of vegetable juice and stir vigorously or blenderize. Sip slowly. Within minutes, your digestive juices will be stimulated and calcium can then be better absorbed and used by your immune system to protect against chemical pollutants that threaten the arthritis breakdown.

YOUR IMMUNE SYSTEM NEEDS ALL MINERALS

Although the preceding have been shown to possess abundantly superior powers of self-immunity, it is important to include all minerals in your food plan. Their actions are interrelated in the body. One mineral is often combined with another to create the needed degree of immunity. A balanced program is important to your immune system.

EATING TIPS FOR STRONGER IMMUNITY

Arm your immune system to fight arthritis virus enemies with some simple nutritional tips:

*Eliminate refined sugar and salt from your diet.
*Avoid excessive fats and processed foods.
*Avoid overcooked foods since they are weak in nutrients.
*Minimize canned foods which are usually cooked twice.
*Avoid deep-fried foods as being too fatty.

With these easy tips, your body will be better able to metabolize minerals and other nutrients and provide a stronger anti-arthritis immune system.

OVERCOMES "AGING ARTHRITIS" AT 56 WITH MINERAL HEALING

Dorothy D. was only 56 when she was diagnosed as having the onset of arthritis. She had recurring pain but the inflammation made her arms and legs so sensitive, she could hardly bear the slightest contact.

Holding a spoon or trying to brush her teeth made her cry out with hurtful pain. She could scarcely do ordinary housework and felt "useless" because her husband and neighboring sister had to do most of it while she looked on with the fear of becoming a helpless invalid.

A relative told Dorothy D. that her so-called "aging arthritis" could be a defect in her immune system. She was diagnosed by an internist who noted she had a deficiency in zinc as well as selenium. This defect was responsible for so-called "aging arthritis" and her other symptoms of chronic weakness and lassitude. She was advised to try a simple "Youth Tonic" that would mineralize her immune system and cast out arthritic invaders.

Dorothy D. mixed the "Youth Tonic" very easily. She said it tasted better than the medication and hoped it would work without side effects. (She had digestive upset because of the drug.) In five days, she felt more energetic. In three weeks, after taking the "Youth Tonic" daily, she was more alert and cheerful. Her inflammation was gone. The pain was hardly more than an occasional tremor which slowly faded away.

She now takes the "Youth Tonic" twice a week and has become younger in mind, body, and spirit. No more "aging arthritis" because of the mineralization of her defense system.

How to Make "Youth Tonic"

In a glass of tomato juice, stir 1 teaspoon of brewer's yeast and one diced garlic clove. Mix thoroughly. Drink slowly.

Immune Boosting Benefits: The zinc of the brewer's yeast combines with the selenium of the garlic and is empowered by the Vitamin C of the tomato juice to supercharge your system with virus-chasing elements. Your immune system is invigorated so that your body casts out so-called "aging" arthritis to make you feel youthfully flexible again.

If you are on a "no nightshade" plan, switch to any other vegetable juice. Cabbage juice is high in Vitamin C which works with the minerals to rebuild the immune system.

FINGERS ARE FLEXIBLE IN ONE WEEK

As a machinist, Matthew E. P. certainly needed the flexibility of his fingers. It was understandable that he became concerned when his middle fingers started to stiffen. His forefingers soon became so hurtfully stiff he could hardly hold a work tool. When his wrists became inflexible and he could scarcely move a small machine, Matthew E. P. decided to seek help.

An orthopedist was consulted. At first, injectable drugs were considered but this was temporarily shelved when he said he always had reactions from medications, even aspirin.

He could have faced surgery but heard the results were often temporary and not always as successful as anticipated. The machinist was in a dilemma. He heard of nutritional therapy and his orthopedist said it would be worth a try. If it did not work, they would have to use surgery which he wanted to avoid under all circumstances.

Matthew E. P. was tested and found to have a borderline selenium-zinc deficiency. It was going to worsen and so would his arthritis. He was given a supplement plan: use brewer's yeast and garlic and also boost his intake of whole grains.

In four days, his fingers were flexible again. By the end of the week, his wrists could move as they did before. He had been "saved" from drugs and surgery, thanks to a nutritional fortification of his immune system.

HOW TO BOOST NUTRITIONAL IMMUNITY

Brewer's Yeast: Little more than a tablespoon a day is usually required for mineralization. Sprinkle in soups, over salads, in stews. Blenderize in fruit or vegetable juices. Use in bread baking, in brown rice pudding, in casseroles, meat or seafood or vegetable entrees.

Garlic: Add a few diced cloves to any raw salad; the pungent taste is offset by grated carrots or a few parsley sprigs. If you cook, use as a replacement for salt (which is antagonistic to the immune system and to be avoided). Add several cloves to soups, stews, vegetable, meat, or fish loaf.

Both of these foods are powerhouses of potent selenium and zinc which your immune system uses as "bricks" against arthritis invaders.

SAVED FROM ARTHRITIS WITH CALCIUM

Helen F. had tried one medication after another for her increasing arthritis. She had such severe low back pain, she was always hunched over, threatening the flexibility of her joints. Drugs had side effects that made her stomach upset and she could scarcely hold food which created even worse malnourishment.

A chiropractor treated her for back trouble and then suggested she take lab tests to detect any defect in her immune system. The report showed she had a marked calcium deficiency.

She was told to boost calcium consumption every day without fail. Helen F. had tried everything so she said this one last hope would not hurt. Indeed not. It helped turn the arthritis tide. The calcium established a stronger immune system so that she soon had minimal discomfort. She soon walked erect, almost ramrod stiff, to show others she had been saved from the crippling disease. "Calcium made me a new person!" she rightfully brags.

CITRUS JUICE EASES MORNING STIFFNESS

A common complaint heard is that of feeling all stiff and painful in the morning. Getting out of bed is often a major chore. Many have found that Vitamin C is a powerful detoxifier of arthritis bacteria and helps create more "get up and go" in the morning.

Grapefruit, orange, or tangerine juice in the morning (singly or in combination) is a dynamic source of Vitamin C when it is most needed. Since this vitamin is water-soluble and not stored in the body, it is often in short supply when you awaken, hence the pain.

The Vitamin C in citrus juice saturates your immune commandos, the white blood cells; it saturates the lymphatic glands which stimulate the immune system. Vitamin C boosts your body's immunity as a whole and has a direct cleansing effect on invading microorganisms such as arthritis antigens.

Minerals are your second line of defense after vitamins in helping to strengthen your immune system to uproot and cast out arthritis invaders and help you enjoy life without this threat!

IN REVIEW

1. Give "youth power" to your immune system with mineralization to cast out arthritis.
2. Zinc, selenium, and calcium are vital for immune fortification and anti-arthritis activity.
3. Absorb calcium more readily into your immune system with the simple apple cider vinegar-honey combo.
4. Dorothy D. overcame "aging" arthritis with mineral healing.
5. The "Youth Tonic" helps your body feel young again in a matter of days, perhaps sooner.
6. Brewer's yeast and garlic are potent immune-boosting foods.
7. Matthew E. P. was saved from drugs and surgery with the use of the two preceding immune-boosting, arthritis-healing foods.
8. Helen F. joins the ranks of winners in the arthritis battle with nutritional therapy. Calcium saved her from crippling arthritis.
9. For early-morning stiffness, citrus juice contains Vitamin C that helps restore flexibility and energy to start your day off with a shout!

8

Pain, Pain Go Away— With a Stronger Immune System

Pain brings more patients to doctors' offices than all other ailments combined. Every year, more than 45 percent of Americans seek medical help for *acute* pain (the short-term discomfort following an injury, infection, or surgery) or *chronic* pain (the suffering that can last a few months or a lifetime).

No one can ever feel or know another's pain. Describing one's pain is exceedingly difficult. You may use words like "throbbing" or "searing." But there is no end to types and degrees of pain. It can come as a dull ache, or a knife-like stab; it can be mild or excruciating, intermittent or constant, transient or prolonged. Pain can be "referred"—felt in a part of the body other than where it began. For the arthritic, pain can be annoying or disabling, no matter how it is described.

WHY PAIN BECOMES SEVERE OR MILD

Pain appears to be worse at night. In the dark and the quiet, when you are alone with your thoughts, you can concentrate on your arthritic pain. What had been mild often turns severe.

Pain's intensity is affected by your overall condition and emotional attitude. Bump your arthritic shoulder one day and you may think nothing of it. Do it again days later, after you've had an emotional upset, and the pain could be much more intense. With a more tranquil mental attitude, your pain could become mild.

HOW PAIN OCCURS IF THE IMMUNE SYSTEM IS WEAK

Pain enters the body because the immune system has become nutritionally deficient to allow this invasion of hurtful substances. (See Figures 8–1 and 8–2.)

When infectious bacteria penetrate the body, cells in the injured tissue release several substances that reduce your body's pain threshold (the level at which a sensation becomes painful): (1) *Histamine* is a major neurotransmitter in the brain, especially in the hippocampus and also throughout the autonomic nervous system; histamine is stored in platelets, mast cells, and basophils; histamine causes dilation of blood vessels and is a hurtful mediator of inflammation. (2) *Prostaglandin* is a hormone-like substance which promotes swelling and inflammation in the area by attracting blood cells to fight infection. (3) *Bradykinin* is one of the most powerful pain-producing substances known; it is a strong polypeptide, a vasodilator, and causes contraction of smooth muscle and plays a hurtful role as a mediator of inflammation.

THE ROUTE OF PAIN IN YOUR BODY

When you develop even the slightest symptom of arthritis because a foreign antigen has penetrated your immune barrier, a chain reaction takes place. Basically, the pain message is carried from the injured area to the spinal cord and from there to the brain.

How Pain Inches Along

These aroused nerve endings send an electrochemical impulse through the nerves to the spinal cord, through which nerve signals from all parts of the body must pass en route to the brain.

THE PAIN PROCESS

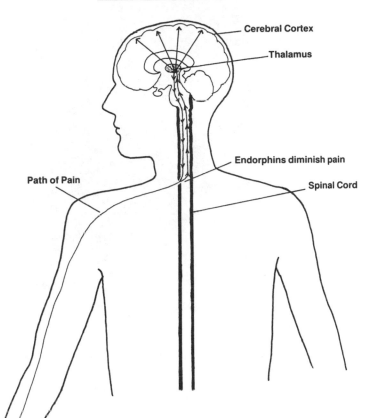

Cerebral Cortex

Thalamus

Endorphins diminish pain

Path of Pain

Spinal Cord

Figure 8-1

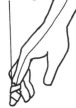

Injured Finger

Pain starts with an injury—the cut or burned finger, for example. Prostaglandins and other body chemicals at the injured area stimulate nerve endings that send the pain message through the spinal cord to the brain. It is at the site of injury that aspirin and non-steroidal, anti-inflammatory drugs are believed to work—diminishing pain by blocking prostaglandin production. In the thalamic region of the brain, the message is consciously recognized as pain, and in the cerebral cortex, the location and severity of the pain are perceived. The signal then descends back down the spinal cord. Within the spinal cord, pain's intensity is thought to be modulated by endorphins and other natural pain-killing chemicals released from the brain to block pain signals.

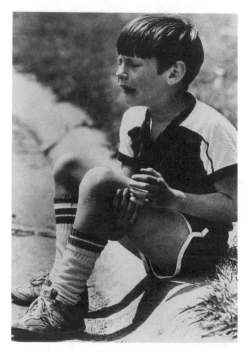

Figure 8–2

Pain can be as innocent and fleeting as that from
a child's scraped knee. But for the millions of sufferers of arthritis, chronic backaches, and headaches, pain can be an agonizing and debilitating
experience.

From the spinal cord, the impulse moves up to the thalamus
region of the brain and to the cerebral cortex. Along the way,
the sensation of arthritic infection is consciously recognized as
pain, and information regarding its intensity and location—and
your emotional reaction to the pain (whether you say "ouch"
or not)—are processed. All of this information is then sent back
down the pain pathways, as further information is ascending.

Depending on how many nerve endings are involved, the
pain can be mild, moderate, or severe. Arthritis, for example,
is a condition in which pain is believed to be linked with
prostaglandin production. The pain message is carried from the
injured area to the spinal cord and from there to the brain.

HOW YOUR IMMUNE SYSTEM SOOTHES PAIN

Your immune system reacts by releasing *endorphins,* natural
pain killers found in the brain. These immune substances inhibit
pain messages by transmitting pain-lessening messages down-

ward from the brain. When your immune system stimulates activation of the brain's endorphin flow, it creates a soothing balm so that pain is eased and even erased.

Location of Natural Pain Killers

The various endorphins seem to be concentrated in the limbic system of the brain which is responsible for your moods and emotions. Endorphin receptors are found in other areas of the brain, which, although not involved in pain perception, do control emotions. These may be brain areas that are responsible for the euphoric effects of drugs.

CAN YOU THINK AWAY YOUR PAIN?

Endorphin receptors have also been located in spinal cord structures that are part of ascending pain pathways. In many studies, it was found that arthritics given placebos (inactive fake pills) feel better. That is, if you *think* you are receiving a pain pill but instead are given a placebo, you may feel better afterward.

This suggests that your brain can somehow activate the production of pain-killing endorphins when you *think and believe* you are receiving an active drug. Endorphins are thereby considered "natural opiates" with morphine or opium-like reactions. Your thoughts often influence endorphin release and pain relaxation.

ACUPUNCTURE AND THE NATURAL OPIATES

Endorphins may also explain why acupuncture, the ancient Chinese healing method, sometimes relieves pain. Through complex nerve pathways, messages of stimulation from the acupuncture needles trigger production of endorphins which then relieve arthritic pain.

Two other methods of relieving pain—the use of electrodes to stimulate peripheral nerves and to stimulate the pain centers of the brain—also may be attributed to stimulation of endorphin secretion. It has also been suggested that hypnosis can provide effective relief from acute pain possibly by similarly promoting endorphin production, but hypnosis is not blocked by narcotic antagonists. It does appear that endorphins are able to relieve pain whether induced by thought or nutrition.

THE NUTRIENT THAT SOOTHES PAIN SWIFTLY

Your immune system needs a little-known but powerful pain-killing nutrient known as *tryptophan.* It is one of the many amino acids and is often found to be in short supply in the arthritic which suggests its need by the immune system.

Tryptophan, Serotonin, Immune Stimulation, Pain Relief

Tryptophan has the ability to initiate the release of a substance called *serotonin* which acts as a neurotransmitter in blocking the pathway of pain. Serotonin is used by your immune system to ease trigger point formation of pain at receptor sites and thereby provide relief of arthritic distress.

Stimulating Tryptophan Activity

Your immune system needs to be nourished with foods containing this amino acid. At the same time, Vitamin B6 and folate (another B-complex member) are needed to stimulate the activity of tryptophan to manufacture the soothing serotonin to ease and minimize arthritic pain.

Food Sources of Tryptophan

Meat, Parmesan and Swiss cheeses, eggs, and almonds are top-notch sources. Milk and yogurt are also good sources of this amino acid. Chicken and turkey are good complete protein sources and also have B-complex nutrients to give a boost to tryptophan production of pain-relieving serotonin.

The immune system of the arthritic often shows a deficiency in tryptophan and this could be a clue to the need for this nutrient in helping to overcome painful symptoms.

TRYPTOPHAN REBUILDS IMMUNE SYSTEM
TO RESIST PAIN

Lewis N. was concerned about becoming addicted to drug-taking for his painful arthritis. He managed most of his duties as a storekeeper but his movements were becoming more and more limited. He had always been an active person; to face the future confined to a chair was more hurtful than his arthritis. Yet drugs made him sweaty, drowsy, and lethargic with slurred speech. He was in a dilemma.

A rheumatologist who frequently emphasized nutritional therapy explained that new tests showed he had markedly low levels of tryptophan. He was told to take 1 gram in supplement form (available at health stores or pharmacies without prescription) to see if it would strengthen his immune system and ease arthritis without the use of drugs.

Desperate, Lewis N. took 1 gram every day. He was advised to take it between meals with a low-protein food such as fruit juice or whole grain bread. *Reason:* Tryptophan is often crowded out by other amino acids in a high-protein meal, preventing it from being absorbed by the immune system to be transported to the brain. After four days, Lewis N. noted his stiffness subsiding. By the end of the sixth day, his arms and legs moved with almost no discomfort. By the start of the ninth day, he could work in the store and even assist loading parcels onto a truck with almost no discomfort. Thanks to tryptophan, his immune system was rebuilt and he was pain-free without the use of drugs.

Benefits of Tryptophan

This amino acid is used by the immune system to release a neurotransmitter, serotonin, to send a response message via the brain downward through the spinal column to "turn off" arthritic pain. This "circuitry" via the immune system detours and casts out pain messages so that serotonin acts as a balm and a soothing contentment for the arthritic.

Feeding Your Immune System a Natural Pain Killer

For many arthritics, the penetration of the immune barrier results in viral attacks upon tissues to trigger pain and/or inflammation and debilitation. Nutritional therapy calls for more than treating the symptoms but also correcting the cause. Tryptophan is able to nourish your immune system, strengthen its fortress, and thereby block future entrance of arthritic invaders. Tryptophan invigorates the T-cells and B-cells to uproot and destroy hurtful infections.

Tryptophan Tonic

In a glass of milk, add 1 teaspoon of brewer's yeast (for B-complex vitamins) and slivered almonds. Blenderize. You now have a potent source of tryptophan *together* with valuable B-complex nutrients that will nourish your immune system to invigorate your brain to release serotonin to tranquilize your arthritic disorder. *Tip:* Remember to drink *between* meals so that there is no competition from other amino acids.

KNEE PAIN VANISHES FOR TROUBLED DANCER

As a former theatre dancer, Rose S. enjoyed her retirement as an instructor for other hopefuls. When she developed arthritic-like pains in her knees and a series of painful spasms while performing simple steps, she felt worried, even frightened.

She wanted a natural method of pain relief because medications, although temporary and not curative, made her feel inflamed and nervous as well as unable to sleep. A young student dancer's father was a homeopathic physician and a believer in natural therapy for the immune system. He took various tests of Rose S. and noted she had markedly low supplies of both tryptophan and Vitamin B6. He told her to take the Tryptophan Tonic every day at 10:00 a.m., and then again at 2:00 p.m. and as a nightcap about one hour before turning in. "Not with meals, please." In seven days, Rose S. could dance with virtually no discomfort. Her immune system had become supercharged with tryptophan, and an outpouring of serotonin created a natural pain relief.

Rose S. was soon more vigorous than the young student dancer, thanks to freeing her knees and other body parts from pain via a tryptophan-invigorated immune system.

Nourish Immune System Easily

Your daily food program should include several of the items listed above as sources of tryptophan. In so doing, the viral invaders can be "knocked out" and eliminated by a strengthened and reconstituted immune system.

TRYPTOPHAN HEALS WHILE YOU SLEEP

This amino acid is so powerful, it can be taken an hour before bedtime to help induce sleep-provoking serotonin and at the same time to stimulate your immune system to release neutrophils and macrophages as well as lymphocytes to uproot and cast out arthritic invaders.

Works While You Sleep

During sleep (made easier by relaxation-inducing serotonin), tryptophan inhibits the pain-causing substances, blocks the reflex pattern, and acts as a natural tranquilizer. You will find that your immune system uses tryptophan to help cleanse away arthritic disturbances while you sleep. Wake up refreshed! Tryptophan helps minimize "morning stiffness" and lethargy! A 1 gram tablet may be all your immune system needs to help heal your arthritis while you sleep.

Tryptophan supplements tend to work most effectively when taken with carbohydrates—starchy foods such as bread, cereal, or potatoes—and not with proteins. As explained, protein foods tend to send in competing amino acids rushing to challenge tryptophan for delivery to the brain.

Do remember to be guided by your health practitioner in the medical use of any amino acid.

MIRACLE AMINO ACID CREATES IMMUNITY AGAINST PAIN

Long regarded only as the building block of protein, new research suggests that phenylalanine may be the brick and mortar of your immune system.

Immunological scientists believe that this amino acid has more value than a building block. It helps soothe your emotions and also strengthens your immune system to reduce painful symptoms.

Phenylalanine, Moods, Arthritis

A viral penetration of the immune system that triggers off painful arthritis can understandably lead to feelings of gloom, even depression. This amino acid reportedly has been able to lift the gloom and make the patient feel better.

Hector C. Sabelli, M.D., a psycho-pharmacologist with the Rush-Presbyterian/St. Luke's Medical Center in Chicago, Illinois, tells us, "In general, phenylalanine is useful as an alternative to anti-depressant drugs in a limited number of cases involving depression of the bipolar type. Bipolar patients can be recognized by the fact that they have recurrent depressions, they tend to be impulsive rather than anxious, and they sleep too much rather than too little."

Dr. Sabelli tells of years of studying the brain chemistry of such patients. "In the body, phenylalanine turns into the active compound, phenylethylamine (PEA), which functions something like an amphetamine. It is a natural amphetamine of the brain.

"The question is, why do some people not form enough phenylethylamine? Is it because they don't get enough in the diet or they don't absorb enough, or is it that they can't transform the phenylalanine into phenylethylamine? We really don't know."

Diet May Be Adequate

Most folks get all the phenylalanine they need in their diet—about 2 grams, says Dr. Sabelli. "There is some of it in all protein foods. In treating depressives, we usually gave 2 to 4 grams a day.

"However, until more is known about phenylalanine, it would be wise for those who suffer from depression to consult their family doctors or psychiatrists first. Too much phenylalanine can function like a mild amphetamine. But for many depressed people, in a clinical setting, this amino acid can help a lot."[1]

Amino Acid Heals Pain

British researchers tested phenylalanine on 22 volunteers who suffered from a wide variety of longstanding ills, from lower back pain to spinal fusion. In seven patients, the phenylalanine, given in 250 milligram daily doses did ease the pain. But for the rest, it had no effect. This suggests that the immune

---

[1] Rush-Presbyterian/St. Luke's Medical Center, Chicago, Illinois, press release, 1986.

system may or may not need this amino acid, and guidance by your health practitioner is advised.[2]

PHENYLALANINE AND PAIN CONTROL

Eric R. Braverman, M.D., with the Brain Bio Center in Rocky Hill, New Jersey, tells us, "Phenylalanine may have the unique ability to block certain enzymes (enkephalinase) in the central nervous system that are normally responsible for degrading (breaking down) natural morphine-like hormones called endorphins and enkephalins. The endorphins and enkephalins act as mild mood elevators and potent analgesics.

Phenylalanine has been suggested to be effective against the chronic pain of osteoarthritis, rheumatoid arthritis, low back pain, joint pains, menstrual cramps, whiplash, and migraine headache."[3]

SAVED FROM SERIOUS PAIN

A 70-year-old man suffered from severe bone pain due to metastatic prostate cancer and his bones were literally being chewed up by his cancer. His pain was resistant to analgesics and DES (diethylstilbesterol—an estrogen drug used for cancer bone pain), the usual treatment for this problem.

Phenylalanine, 1.5 grams in the morning and another 1.5 grams in the evening, brought this patient's terrible pain under control.[4]

HELPS DEFUSE PAIN THREAT

This noteworthy amino acid thereby appears to have the power to release endorphins and defuse the pain threat because of the hurtful histamine, prostaglandin, and bradykinin neurotransmitters.

---

[2] *Advances in Pain Research and Therapy,* New York, Volume 5, 1983, pp. 305–308.

[3] Eric R. Braverman, M.D., "The Healing Nutrients Within," Keats Publishing Inc., New Canaan, Connecticut, p. 39, 1987.

[4] K. Budd, M.D., *Advances in Pain Research and Therapy,* New York, Volume 5, 1983, pp. 305–308.

Food Sources: Like most amino acids, phenylalanine is highly concentrated in high-protein foods. These include wheat germ, granola, oat flakes, ricotta cheese, cottage cheese, chicken, and wild game.

Immune Boosting Remedy: Mid-morning, try an *Amino Acid Pain Stopper*—in an 8-ounce container of plain cottage cheese, stir in 1 teaspoon wheat germ, 1 teaspoon oat flakes, and combine thoroughly. Eat slowly with a spoon. Your metabolism uses the phenylalanine in this *Amino Acid Pain Stopper* to fortify your immune system. At the same time, the amino acid is dispatched to your brain to release substances that act as endorphins . . . they dilute the hurtful neurotransmitters and participate in their removal from the body. In a short time, thanks to phenylalanine power, your immune system will shield your body against arthritic pain.

Caution: Phenylalanine is not to be used by those who have phenylketonuria, an inborn error of this amino acid. The PKU condition, as it is called, has an excess of this amino acid and additional amounts are inadvisable. If you have PKU, follow your health practitioner's advice with regards to amino acid intake.

RELIEVING ARTHRITIS WITH PHENYLALANINE

Arnold Fox, M.D., in his research, tells of starting his arthritis patients on this amino acid program: 375 milligrams with breakfast, 375 milligrams with lunch, 375 milligrams with dinner.

"I instruct my patients to have regular meals: breakfast at 8 a.m., lunch at noon, and dinner between 5 and 6 p.m., in the evening. Phenylalanine should be taken with the meal, or within an hour after completing the meal. I prefer it to be taken five minutes after the meal. On the third day, if no pain relief has occurred, I generally have them increase the dosage to 750 milligrams with breakfast, 750 milligrams with lunch, and 750 milligrams with dinner.

"If my patients have trouble sleeping at night because the amino acid gives them a feeling of excitement or energy, I have them cut the dinner dose in half. I tell my patients to stay with it—give it a chance to work.

"My observation has been that it takes anywhere from two days to three weeks for phenylalanine to take effect. It may take as long as four to six weeks, so I encourage my patients not to get discouraged. Phenylalanine is not fast-acting like aspirin. It takes at least two days to have effect. Give it a chance to work.

"When they have felt really good for a full week, I have my patients stop taking it and wait for the arthritis symptoms to recur. They go on an alternating schedule, taking phenylalanine until they feel good for a full week, then not taking it until the symptoms reappear, and so on. Many of my patients only use phenylalanine one out of every three or four weeks. Patients are encouraged to adjust their dosage in consultation with their physician."[5]

THE IMMUNE BOOSTING ANTI-ARTHRITIS
AMINO ACID

Give your immune system the nutritional power to resist arthritis pain with the use of a little-known amino acid—histidine. While you make some histidine in your body, most is obtained from the diet. Yet it has been found that many arthritis sufferers have a deficiency of this amino acid and this could be a reason for the discomfort and pain of the condition.

Eric R. Braverman, M.D., tells us, "Of the 22 reported studies on amino acids in rheumatoid arthritis, histidine is the only amino acid consistently found to be in short supply.

"Eight of the studies show low histidine levels in blood serum. Low histidine levels are also found in arthritic synovial fluid—the transparent, viscid, lubricating fluid secreted by joint membranes.

"These observations led to the first clinical trials of histidine therapy. Rheumatoid arthritis patients frequently have low blood histidine levels because histidine is removed more rapidly than

---

[5] Arnold Fox, M.D., *DLPA to End Chronic Pain and Depression*, Pocket Books, 1985, pp. 117–118.

average from their blood, as shown by abnormally low levels in histidine tolerance tests."

Histidine Therapy Is Healing

D. A. Gerber, M.D., of Downstate Medical Center in Brooklyn, N.Y., tells of treating several rheumatoid arthritis patients with 1 gram or more daily and found improvement in grip strength and walking ability. Only two out of the eight rheumatoid arthritis patients tested by Dr. Gerber showed histidine levels of over 1.30 milligrams per 100 milliliters of blood. Patients that had high sed rates (erythrocyte sedimentation rate—a marker of inflammation) and great difficulty in walking responded best to histidine therapy.[6]

Feed Histidine to Immune System

Although no definite daily intake for histidine has been established, many experts suggest a rule-of-thumb rate at about 10 milligrams per day. Good sources would be wheat germ, cheese, ricotta cheese, rolled oats, chicken, turkey, and wild game.

HELP YOUR IMMUNE SYSTEM NIP PAIN IN THE BUD

Your immune system needs nutritional support to build resistance against the invasion of enemy substances that are responsible for arthritic pain; namely, histamine, prostaglandin, and bradykinin. Your immune system is able to send forth antibodies via the T- and B-lymphocyte network to block the formation of prostaglandins, for example, thus reducing inflammation and pain. These immune-released antibodies also inhibit prostaglandins and bradykinins, and this will decrease pain sensations.

Your immune system's antibodies prompt the release of enkephalins, endorphins, and dynorphins which are opiate-like compounds that work on the receptor sites in the brain.

The immune-released antibodies help block pain directly at the sight of the arthritic hurt; they also block pain signals

---

[6] *Journal of Rheumatology,* 4:40–45, 1977.

that have already entered the central nervous system. They prevent the transfer of pain signals from the dorsal horn (close to back of body) to the thalamus in the brain. These same antibodies alert your pain-suppressing system and help relieve and block out arthritic pain. The goal is to stimulate your immune system to release antibodies that lock into specific "receptor sites" within the pain centers and provide relaxation and comfort in a short time.

Nutrients are an important part of the plan to stimulate immune-building responses to release antibodies that promote freedom from arthritic pain. Help your immune system make the hurt go away!

IN REVIEW

1. A weakness in your immune system allows release of histamine, prostaglandin, and bradykinin antigens that cause arthritic pain.
2. In some situations, if you *think* you are being healed, you can turn off the pain with mind power.
3. Soothe pain swiftly with a little-known immune boosting amino acid. It works as effectively as a chemical.
4. Lewis N. stimulated his immune system with tryptophan and overcame painful stiffness without the use of drugs.
5. A Tryptophan Tonic creates an immune response to "knock out" arthritic hurt.
6. Rose S. overcame crippling knee pain with the Tryptophan Tonic.
7. Phenylalanine was used by physicians to boost the immune system and control pain.
8. A 70-year-old man had "terrible pain" that a doctor brought under control with the use of this amino acid.
9. A noted physician suggests a simple phenylalanine program to relieve arthritic pain.
10. A leading physician brought arthritis under control with the use of histidine, a little-known but powerful immune boosting nutrient.

9

How Anti-Oxidants Free You from the Painful Grip of Arthritis

The newer knowledge of immunity against arthritis recognizes that the condition is often sparked because of microscopic chemical fragments in the body dubbed "free radicals" or "oxygen free radicals."

Basically, free radicals are highly unstable chemicals found in the body and are believed to develop as a byproduct of metabolism. For food to be metabolized, oxygen must pass through the mitochondria (a chemically active pocket in the cell). Free radicals are the waste products left behind.

Although most free radicals automatically leave the body after participating in metabolic reactions, some remain and their activities are controlled by enzymes.

Arthritis and Free Radicals

Immunologists have found that some of these unstable chemicals accumulate and do arthritic injury by interfering with the workings of healthy cells. As evidence, some researchers point to the body's accumulation of lipofuscin, or age pigments, an end product of free radical interactions.

103

Immune System, Free Radicals

Researchers believe that free-radical-caused arthritis results in a faulty immune system. Basically, there is a decrease in lymphocyte (white blood cells) response to antigens (foreign elements which spark arthritis and other conditions). If free radical injury could be lessened, the immune system may be able to remain stronger and not only resist arthritis but also help correct and eliminate its presence.

Scientists have found that one of the primary causes of the weakness in the immune system is a loss of T-cell function. T-cells are one of two broad classifications of lymphocytes which produce antibodies to fight arthritis and other illnesses. T-cells are formed in the bone marrow but are eventually housed in the thymus, an organ of the lymph system located at the back of the neck. They take their name, T-cells, from their relationship to the thymus.

ANTI-OXIDANTS BOOST IMMUNE SYSTEM FUNCTION

In one reported situation, scientists measured the effect of anti-oxidants (substances believed to inhibit free radical reactions) on the formation and propagation of free radicals.

The researchers fed subjects anti-oxidants and noted there was greater immune functioning and reduction of free-radical damage so there was less risk of arthritis.

How Anti-Oxidants Protect Against Arthritis

These substances stimulate the immune system to survey cells throughout the body and destroy those which appear threatening or foreign. The anti-oxidants energize your immune system to recognize "self" (cells or organs or other body parts) and "non-self" (cells of a grafted organ or an abnormal cell). If there is a nutritional deficiency, this ability to distinguish between "self" and "non-self" weakens. At times it can even turn on itself, producing autoimmune reactions such as those which result in rheumatoid arthritis.

Anti-oxidants are nutrients found in certain foods that appear to counteract this deficiency-caused weakening of the immune system.

Robert C. Atkins, M.D., prominent New York City physician tells us, "Some of the same biochemical changes that affect the arterial wall in atherosclerosis are also evident in arthritic joints. Free radicals, which are highly reactive, unstable molecules with unattached electrons, and which by their chemical nature are obliged to react immediately with one of the body's normal chemicals, have been shown to initiate damage to the joint membrane in acute rheumatoid arthritis."

What Is the Value of Anti-Oxidants?

Dr. Atkins says, "As is true in heart disease, perhaps the most damaging free radicals are peroxides. These unstable chemicals are the results of a sort of molecular supersaturation with free oxygen. Their tendency is to oxidize any molecule they contact."

Nutritional Immunity

"Much of the benefit derived from the nutritional anti-oxidants Vitamin C and Vitamin E and the mineral selenium can be attributed to their ability to prevent peroxidation damage."

Superoxide Dismutase

"We can carry the principle of anti-oxidation one step further by using the same enzyme maintained in our bodies' own cells to protect them against peroxidation. Superoxide dismutase (SOD) is an enzyme residing within our cells for the purpose of inactivating the peroxide radicals. Much basic biochemical research has made peroxide 'suspect number one' as the chemical that initiates the rheumatoid process.

"Since SOD has become clinically available, I have been using it on my arthritic patients, and it seems to work. (Although I always wonder if any enzymes will maintain their biologic effectiveness when taken by mouth and then having to pass through the highly acid stomach contents.) But it requires a lot—usually more than a dozen pills taken throughout the day are needed to get any results."

Nutritional Fortification

"The most intriguing treatment, nutritionally, may well be that there are several superoxide dismutases, some which require copper and zinc to be active and others which require either manganese or iron. All of these minerals (with the possible exception of iron) have been reported effective in treating arthritis. Of these, the most promising is copper."[1]

FREE RADICALS: IMMUNE DESTROYING MOLECULES

The most important element in the air you breathe—oxygen—may not be as innocent as it seems. Oxygen is vital to human life. However, some forms of it can hurt the living tissue and immune system. Oxygen free radicals are these by-products of normal body metabolism that can destroy the immune system or impair its ability to function. (See Figures 9–1 and 9–2.)

Why do free radicals build up? Some causes include tissue and organ injury, inflammation, cancer, cardiovascular disease, and aging.

Free radicals are potentially destructive, reactive, with a special affinity for lipids (fats), proteins, and nucleic acids (DNA and RNA backbone).

Free radicals penetrate the immune barrier when a molecule gains an extra electron (a negatively charged particle). They are hurtful to the immune system because they can: (1) damage lipids or fats within the cells; (2) fragment DNA strands, producing genetic mutations; (3) damage proteins, resulting in the loss of biological activity; (4) destroy important body cells; (5) produce inflammation; (6) cause severe injury or cell death in the lungs; (7) damage blood vessels; (8) decrease the activity and availability of neurotransmitters (brain chemicals that carry messages from one nerve cell to the next).

Inflammation, Rheumatoid Arthritis

There is ample evidence that oxygen radicals are involved in the inflammatory response. During an arthritic inflammatory reaction, a large number of cells called phagocytes can ingest

---

[1] *Dr. Atkins' Nutrition Breakthrough* by Robert C. Atkins, M.D., Bantam Books, Inc., 1981, pp. 172–173.

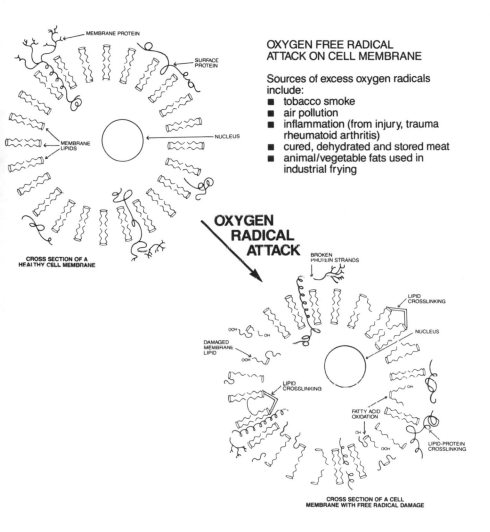

OXYGEN FREE RADICAL
ATTACK ON CELL MEMBRANE

Sources of excess oxygen radicals
include:
- tobacco smoke
- air pollution
- inflammation (from injury, trauma rheumatoid arthritis)
- cured, dehydrated and stored meat
- animal/vegetable fats used in industrial frying

Oxygen radicals are extremely reactive and short-lived by-products of body metabolism capable of damaging living tissue. Oxygen free radicals can attack cell membranes, causing damage to lipids and proteins. They cause oxidation of lipids (lipid peroxides—fats chemically altered by oxygen radicals that are unable to perform normal cellular functions). This process can impair a cell's ability to function or even destroy it.

COURTESY—THE UPJOHN COMPANY

Figure 9–1

SOME CONDITIONS LINKED TO OXYGEN RADICALS

Conditions	Number of New Cases In the United States per Year
CARDIOVASCULAR DISEASES	63,400,000*
RHEUMATOID ARTHRITIS	2,100,000**
CENTRAL NERVOUS SYSTEM:	
HEAD TRAUMA	450,000
SPINAL CORD INJURY	10,000
STROKE	500,000
EMPHYSEMA	191,000
CANCER	930,000
ADULT RESPIRATORY DISTRESS SYNDROME	150,000
MAJOR ORGAN TRANSPLANTS (does not include tissue transplants)	38,541
INFLAMMATION	—
AGING	—

*Estimated total number of people with cardiovascular diseases as of 1984.
**Estimated total number of people with rheumatoid arthritis as of 1986.

Excessive production of oxygen radicals—highly reactive and unstable by-products of oxygen metabolism—are tied to tissue damage in a variety of conditions. Scientists are developing novel therapeutic strategies to mop up or "scavenge" oxygen radicals and bolster enzymes that convert radicals to less toxic substances.

Figure 9–2

microorganisms or other foreign particles that invade the site of injury or infection. Phagocytes release oxygen radicals that aid in digesting foreign particles.

In some inflammatory arthritis conditions, the body seems unable to recognize foreign particles from its own cells. An example is rheumatoid arthritis. The lack of recognition sets the phagocytes in motion around the joints, leading to the release of oxygen radicals and subsequent joint damage. With the use of nutritional anti-oxidants, an abundance of neutrophils (cleansers) will minimize the radicals and reduce the number of inflammatory cells found in tissue surrounding the joints.

Avoid These Immune Threats

Normal metabolism is not the only source of immune-threatening free radicals. Air pollutants; pesticides; tobacco smoke; X-ray and ultraviolet radiation; cured, dehydrated, and stored meats, as well as fats used in frying at very high temperatures— all trigger the accumulation of free radicals that weaken the immune system, badly injure cells, and render the body vulnerable to arthritic infection.

Be especially careful to avoid carbon monoxide, nitric oxide, unburnt hydrocarbons, and ozone, all of which can penetrate your immune barriers and weaken your defense system.

HOW NUTRITION BOOSTS IMMUNE RESISTANCE AND RECOVERY

A group of nutrients will help your body strengthen the immune system and minimize the hurt of the free radicals. These nutrients comprise the anti-oxidant family. Namely, they will: (1) convert cellular oxidants to water and oxygen (non-radical) through the action of various enzymatic defenses, and (2) reduce the concentration of hurtful free radicals by the action of scavengers or cleansers.

Protective anti-oxidant molecules capable of "scavenging" oxygen radicals include beta-carotene, Vitamin C, Vitamin E, and superoxide dismutase or SOD. These nutrients "mop up" free radicals, change them into weaker, less hurtful substances, and rebuild your immune system.

Anti-oxidants inhibit lipid peroxidation, an immune-destroying condition linked to arthritis. Basically, lipid peroxides are fats that become chemically altered because of free-radical attack. They threaten your immune system by releasing potent chemicals that damage the tissues, reduce blood flow, hinder metabolism, and interfere with other cellular functions.

Your immune system can protect you against arthritis with nutritional fortification via the anti-oxidants.

FOUR ANTI-OXIDANTS THAT PROTECT AGAINST ARTHRITIS HURT

To help take the "hurt" out of arthritis and wash out invading free radicals, four anti-oxidants are needed by your immune system.

#1—Beta-Carotene

Arthritis Healing Benefit: Beta-carotene (a meatless source of Vitamin A) releases molecules that distribute cell-washing phagocytes; a stimulation of T-cell production dispatches neutrophils to digest foreign particles and cool off the inflammatory cells found in areas around the joints.

Sources: Sweet potatoes, carrots, spinach, cantaloupe, broccoli, apricots, and peaches.

#2—Vitamin C

Arthritis Healing Benefit: A water-soluble anti-oxidant that penetrates the fluid compartments of a cell to cause a breakdown in the defense system and render the body vulnerable to arthritis. It works together with Vitamin E to boost its active cleansing form.

Sources: Citrus fruits such as oranges, grapefruits, tangerines, lemons, limes, green peppers, broccoli, papayas, Brussels sprouts, cantaloupe, and cabbage.

#3—Vitamin E

Arthritis Healing Benefit: A fat-soluble vitamin that penetrates lipid membranes; it removes the dangerous unpaired electron from an oxygen radical. This transfer of electrons reduces a free radical or lipid peroxide to a less toxic form.

Vitamin E protects the cell by becoming oxidized itself, thereby sparing surrounding healthy tissue.

Sources: Wheat germ oil, sunflower seed, raw wheat germ, sunflower seed oil, almonds, pecans, hazelnuts, whole grain breads and cereals, and baked goods.

#4—Selenium

Arthritis Healing Benefit: Unique in being able to form an anti-oxidant enzyme known as glutathione which enhances the immune system and helps minimize the hurt of free-radical attack. Selenium is needed to neutralize the free radicals by pairing up their electrons to protect the body's cells.

Sources: Seafood, whole grain breads and cereals, broccoli, cabbage, and onions. *Note:* The amounts of selenium in foods may vary according to the level of the mineral in the soils where they were produced. In general, soils in the west contain more selenium than those in the east.

Free Yourself from Arthritis with Anti-Oxidants

Because there is so much oxygen in body tissues and because oxygen tends to form highly reactive radicals by gaining extra electrons (negative charges), many of your cells contain these potential saboteurs to your health and well-being. You need an ample daily supply of anti-oxidants as a means of defending against these hurtful and immune-destroying free radicals. Include them in your daily food program and you will strengthen your immune system and be free of arthritis.

VITAMINS "WASH OUT" ARTHRITIS PAIN

Getting out of a chair caused Noreen R. to silently cry out with arthritic pain. It was agonizing at times for her to reach into high shelves or stretch upward. As for bending, she had to bite down hard to avoid weeping because of the shooting pains. She had long ago been compelled to give up a lucrative supervisor's job because of her creeping limited movements. She felt "imprisoned" in her own body!

A medical supply salesman in her neighborhood had once been the victim of near-crippling arthritis himself and overcame his condition by "washing out" hurtful free radicals. He had been diagnosed as having this immune system defect and was told to take all four anti-oxidants through improved diet. He told Noreen R. that she, too, could have a breakdown in her immune system and suggested she boost intake of anti-oxidant foods.

Desperate for any straw of help, Noreen R. boosted consumption of as many anti-oxidant foods as possible that were prime sources of beta-carotene, Vitamins C and E, and also selenium. Progress was slow for two weeks when she was told to avoid tobacco smoke (her husband and older son were heavy smokers and henceforth forbidden to bring these health threats into the house). She was also to eliminate any processed or "cured" meats and to avoid any type of fried foods. By the end of the fifth week, her back was more flexible. In seven weeks, she had only minimal spasms when stretching or bending and was soon so limber, she was able to regain her former job. The anti-oxidants had been able to "wash out" the free radicals to the extent that the oxidation was eased and her immune system was strengthened to resist arthritis.

She was so overjoyed, she celebrated with friends, family, and the medical supply salesman who had helped her "escape" from the prison of arthritis via anti-oxidant immune stimulation.

HOW TO NOURISH YOUR IMMUNE SYSTEM WITH ARTHRITIS-HEALING ANTI-OXIDANTS

Because there are 100 (or more) forms of arthritis, it is important to supply your body with a number of anti-oxidants to help provide as many antidotes as possible. Not every program works the same for every person. Arthritis has many faces. If you, for example, have standard rheumatoid arthritis, a neighbor with the same diagnosed condition may be in more discomfort or less.

You may have more or less free-radical injury than your neighbor. Your immune system may be stronger or weaker than that of your neighbor. In planning an arthritis-fighting program with anti-oxidant foods at the top of the list, you would do well to supply your body with a variety of these nutrients. As symptoms subside, you will be able to make any necessary adjustments. Your body will tell you whether you need more or less of the anti-oxidants.

Basically, you will help keep free radicals under control and also reduce formation of lipid peroxides which are known for causing injury, with these immune-invigorating improvements in your lifestyle:

1. Avoid tobacco smoke in all its forms.

2. Keep as far away from air pollution as possible. Make frequent trips to the country or any fresh air region to cleanse your system and keep free radicals from multiplying due to pollution.

3. Any injury, however slight, should be properly treated. A hurt from a fall may not cause breakage but will injure tissue and lead to formation of free radicals that could multiply to hurt your immune system.

4. Foods should be freshly prepared. Say *NO* to anything that is fried, dehydrated, or cured. If you have no alternative, use them at a minimum. It is best to avoid any stored animal or vegetable fats.

5. If possible, avoid pesticides through inhalation or ingestion since they can give rise to cellular breakdown and a weakness in the immune system. These chemicals hinder the cleansing process of metabolism and other immune-building cellular functions in your tissues.

6. X-rays and ultraviolet radiation should also be minimized. They can play havoc with your immune system and give rise to destructive, mismatched electrons and hurtful free radicals.

7. It may be easier said than done to avoid any cured, dehydrated, and stored meats as well as fats used in frying at very high temperatures. These all add to the growth of free radicals that can badly damage cells and give rise to arthritis. Eat out a lot? Select restaurants that use more healthful methods of cooking such as baking, broiling, boiling. Do the same at home!

With these immune-invigorating improvements, your lifestyle will be all the stronger and you will have a resistant shield against hurtful free radicals.

ANTI-OXIDANT BREAKFAST FOR FLEXIBLE BODY AND MIND

Invigorate your immune system with "cell washing" anti-oxidants so you will have flexibility of body and mind from early morning until late hours: A fruit salad with chunks of peaches, cantaloupe, and apricots; a whole-grain cereal sprinkled with Vitamin C powder and raisins; several citrus fruit wedges; enjoy whole grain muffins; a glass of citrus juice or a mixed vegetable juice.

Benefit: These foods are prime sources of valuable anti-oxidants that work as radical cleansers. You'll be able to feel more energetic in body and mind with this immune invigoration.

IMMUNE-BOOSTING FOODS—ANTI-OXIDANT CELL CLEANSING

*Replace commercial desserts with fresh fruits in any combination, but emphasize citrus for important Vitamin C.

*A baked sweet potato is a terrific source of beta-carotene and can often be used as an entree together with a raw salad made of shredded cabbage, green pepper, and broccoli sprinkled with slivered almonds and pecans.

*Replace caffeine-containing beverages which could break down defenses against arthritis with the use of a variety of fruit and vegetable juices, rich in anti-oxidants.

*Seafood is a great source of needed selenium which is one of the most powerful anti-oxidant foods needed by your immune system. Enjoy seafood several times a week.

*Drench your immune system with anti-oxidants by enjoying lightly steamed broccoli, spinach, carrots, and cabbage as a healthful salad. A fresh papaya is another great anti-oxidant food.

*On any green salad, sprinkle wheat germ and sunflower seeds for a piquant taste along with onion rings. A bit of wheat germ oil adds to the palatability. Anti-oxidants flourish in these foods and are needed to energize your immune system to ease and erase arthritic symptoms.

With these basic guidelines, you can tastefully feed yourself and still maintain a healthy immune system.

NIPS ARTHRITIS IN THE BUD WITH ANTI-OXIDANT FOODS

A family history of arthritis made George Z. worry when his fingers became stiff and he would feel tingling heat and sensitive inflammation around his knees and legs. Was he destined to follow in his arthritic family's footsteps?

A rheumatologist in his neighborhood was known for using "holistic" or "total body" healing methods and did offer hope to George Z. He was given a thorough nutritional assessment to reveal that he was largely deficient in Vitamin E and selenium. He had an excessive amount of free radicals. He was given prescribed supplements of these nutrients. George Z. was put on a simple nutritional program—avoid fried foods, no cured, dehydrated, or stored meats, no stored animal or vegetable fats for frying.

George Z. was told to use fresh wheat germ oil for baking or broiling and also on salads. At the same time, he increased consumption of the spectrum of anti-oxidant foods listed above.

These four anti-oxidant food groups so bolstered his immune system that within six weeks, his arthritis was about gone. His rheumatologist took another test to see if he had fewer free radicals and a stronger immune system.

Did he inherit the arthritis or a nutritionally weak immune system? George Z. had overcome so-called heredity with a well-nourished immune system!

YOU *CAN* LIVE *WITHOUT* ARTHRITIS

With the use of anti-oxidants, you can detoxify free radicals and give your immune system the ability to "wash out" your hurtful waste products. With these nutritional invigorators, you *can* be free of arthritis and enjoy good health of body and mind.

IN REVIEW

1. A probable clue to the cause of arthritis is the presence of excessive free radicals in the system, responsible for the hurtful symptoms because of a weakened immune system.

2. Anti-oxidants found in everyday foods help protect against molecular supersaturation with rancid oxygen.

3. Guard against threats to your immunity via air pollution, environmental assaults, and processed meat products.

4. Check the list of the four basic anti-oxidants and their easily available foods.

5. Noreen R. used anti-oxidant vitamins to "wash out" her arthritis pain in a short time. She felt released from the prison of arthritis.

6. Follow the seven immune-invigorating lifestyle improvement steps to a stronger immune system, free of arthritis-causing free radicals.

7. Nourish your immune system with anti-oxidant suggestions as listed.

8. George Z. avoided so-called "inherited arthritis" with an anti-oxidant program.

10

How Seafood
Washes Away Arthritic Pain

You hurt when your immune system is unable to cope with an outpouring of a hormone-like substance called prostaglandin. It would be easy to say that all you need do is block prostaglandin and you will no longer have arthritic pain. But this substance has several faces. It is needed to regulate vital metabolic processes throughout your body. You could hardly survive without it. The key is to balance the outpouring so that you do not have too much of a good thing.

Although there are over 30 known prostaglandins, they occur in nature basically in three major series (named series one, two, and three, based on the number of chemical double bonds). Of these there are two members (of the "two" series) that are important to your immune system and freedom from arthritic pain.

Looking at Prostaglandins

The "bad guy" is called thromboxane which circulates with the platelets and tightens your blood vessels to cause problems. The "good guy" is called prostacyclin which protects against this constriction and maintains free circulation.

You have these two biochemical substances with opposing action. Compare it to having a devil on one shoulder and an angel on the other.

That is, you have two parallel systems of prostaglandins, both slightly different in structure. You need to release more of the "good guy prostacyclin" or PGE1, as it is called, to help soothe your pain and less of the "bad guy thromboxane" or PGE2.

Soothe Pain with Seafood

Immunologists have reported that certain types of seafood contain a beneficial substance identified as eicosapentaenoic acid or EPA, which promotes PGE1 but controls PGE2.

OMEGA-3 FISH OILS LUBRICATE YOUR JOINTS

Omega-3 fatty acids are a sort of polyunsaturated fat found in greatest concentration in fatty cold-water fish. The EPA in these fatty acids encourages the production of the beneficial "good guy prostacyclin" or PGE1. It develops in cells which occupy the lining of arteries.

Fish oils with the EPA content helps block some inflammatory processes. EPA interferes with the production of hurtful "bad guy thromboxane" and prevents the release of other substances known as *leukotrienes* which give you all-too-familiar inflammation.

Speaking simply, Omega-3 fatty acids produce "good" prostaglandins, protect against inflammation, and shield you from pain. In some rheumatoid arthritics, there is a significant reduction in tender joints and fatigue when consuming these fish oils.

Omega-3 fish oils also contain docosahexaenoic acid or DHA which helps create a balance of prostaglandin release to immunize you against inflammation and hurt.

FISH OILS AS TREATMENT FOR ARTHRITIS

Several studies have suggested that certain fish oils may reduce the symptoms of rheumatoid arthritis and possibly systemic lupus erythematosus. Scientists conducting the studies believe that the fish oils interfere with the process of inflammation, a key factor in the condition.

How Fish Oils Are Healing

Specifically, the scientists have found that these fish oils contain substances called Omega-3 fatty acids which reduce the body's production of another substance called arachidonic acid. This substance plays an important role in causing inflammation of joints and other tissues.

Arachidonic acid is made from fatty acids which are found in a normal diet. But the Omega-3 fatty acids in fish oil are different. When they take the place of the body's normal fatty acids, they can prevent the body from using arachidonic acid and, thus, inhibit painful inflammation.

STUDIES OFFER HOPE FOR ARTHRITIS HEALING WITH FISH OILS

Daily consumption of fish oil reportedly led to welcome improvement in the symptoms of rheumatoid arthritis patients in clinical tests.

Richard I. Sperling, M.D., a Harvard University Instructor of Medicine, announces, "Our trial, although it was relatively small, shows evidence that fish oil does have promise for inflammatory disease."

Dr. Sperling and his colleagues examined different groups of patients and noted that fish oils protected the body from "inflammatory products." Namely, the Omega-3 fish oils helped inhibit the release of leukotriene, the cause of much painful swelling.

Fewer Tender Joints

In treating other patients with active arthritis, Dr. Sperling reports the use of Omega-3 fish oils was helpful. "We saw a suppression of inflammatory products. The patients definitely felt better. They had fewer tender joints and reported less pain. Other studies will follow this up. Right now, we know we can at least biochemically alter the generation of inflammatory products in cells."[1]

---

[1] *Arthritis and Rheumatism,* 25:133, 1983.

Helps Rheumatoid Arthritis

Joel M. Kremer, M.D., of Albany Medical College, an Associate Professor of Medicine, and his colleagues, reported on a 40-patient, placebo-controlled, double-blind, cross-over study. They gave 15 MaxEpa capsules daily to 20 patients for 14 weeks. The patients continued their normal diets with the only difference being the MaxEpa supplement.

At the same time another group of 20 arthritis patients took the same number of placebo capsules. After the 14-week period, all 40 patients began a 4-week washout period in which they took no MaxEpa or placebo. The groups were then "crossovered"; i.e., each group then took the capsules formerly taken by the other group for 14 weeks. Another 4-week washout period followed. Thirty-three patients completed the clinical trial.

Dr. Kremer reports, "Those taking fish oil had only about half the number of tender joints as they had prior to the study, and about half as many as the patients taking the placebo. The benefit vanished during the washout period." They also add that the fish oils slowed the onset of fatigue.

The fish oils helped balance the release of substances so there was less incidence of discomfort. Dr. Kremer reports, "We saw a significant correlation between the drop in leukotriene B4 and the decrease in the number of tender joints.

"Those receiving the EPA supplement were not in as much pain; their joints were less tender and they made it through the day longer before fatigue set in." He adds, "We also found benefits four weeks after the fish oil was discontinued."

Fish Helps Arthritis Swim Away

As a means of boosting the immune system to resist inflammation, fish oils are important. Dr. Kremer tells us, "It is irrefutable that eating more fish is a healthy step for any person, arthritis or not. Researchers do have more well-developed evidence that fish oil can be a key step in lowering cholesterol and fighting cardiovascular trouble such as atherosclerosis and heart attacks.

"In our studies, the doses of fish oil given were roughly equal to a salmon dinner or a can of sardines.

"If you've got arthritis now, you can use traditional therapy for relief and also continue to eat more fish. It certainly won't hurt and may help your inflammation.

"Then look to the next few years for a possible new inflammatory disease treatment—fish oil."[2]

BEFORE YOU CONSIDER SUPPLEMENTS

Fish oil supplements are available but they have not been carefully studied with regard to long term effects and safety. Potential risks, such as prolonged bleeding or reduced clotting time, need to be considered. A prudent approach may be the most appropriate one.

How much Omega-3's should the arthritic be consuming? That has not been established and moderation should be the order of the day. Experts suggest consumption of 4 to 6 ounces of fish twice a week as a good way to stimulate your immune system and ease the shock waves of hurtful prostaglandins. Salmon and mackerel are considered among the best sources of Omega-3 fatty acids and should be consumed regularly.

FISH OILS, ARTHRITIS, IMMUNITY

Richard S. Panush, M.D., of the University of Florida College of Medicine in Gainesville, tells us:

"The use of diet to treat rheumatic disease (arthritis) is an important topic in contemporary clinical immunology and has been identified by the rheumatologists as among the major clinical advances of the future."

It has also been noted that some food may aggravate the symptoms of rheumatoid arthritis. At the 1986 meeting of the American Rheumatism Association, 5 percent of all people with rheumatic disease were estimated to have an immunologic sensitivity to some foods.

Based on preliminary evidence from animal and human studies, Dr. Panush suggested two possible mechanisms that need not be mutually exclusive:

---

[2] *Clinical Research,* 33:A778, 1985.

1. Food antigens might provoke hypersensitive responses or food allergies.

2. Dietary changes might alter immune and inflammatory responses, thus affecting the symptoms.

In an animal experiment, for example, inflammatory synovitis (swelling of the synovial membrane of a joint) occurred when cow's milk was substituted for water.

Also, "challenge testing" has proven that people can suffer delayed reactions—up to 48 hours—after ingesting an offending food. After a fasting period, people are "challenged" with a suspect food given in capsule form.

It is very likely that as one food could trigger an arthritis reaction, another food may cause the condition to become soothed. This could be the situation with fish oils.[3]

Food Sources of EPA and DHA
Omega-3 Fatty Acids

FOOD	TOTAL FAT GRAMS	OMEGA-3 FATTY ACIDS GRAMS
(All 3½ ounces, raw)		
Bass, striped	2.3	0.8
Bluefish	6.5	1.2
Hake, silver	2.6	0.6
Herring, Atlantic	9.0	1.7
Mackerel, Atlantic	13.9	2.6
Mullet	4.4	1.1
Pompano, Florida	9.5	0.6
Sablefish	15.3	1.5
Salmon, sockeye	8.6	1.3
Shark	1.9	0.5
Swordfish	2.1	0.2
Tuna, bluefin	6.6	1.6

AGONIZING PAIN EASED WITH FISH OILS

It started with a feeling of numbness in Bill D.'s toes and a feeling that his shoes were uncomfortable. Everytime he stood, it felt as if he were on rocks. Then it progressed to the point

---

[3] *Annals of Internal Medicine,* April, 1987.

where he was troubled with extremely sharp pains, as if someone took a board studded with needles and raked it across the tops of his toes.

First he would get one pain, then another. A few seconds later, more pain. He never knew when it would strike again. Bill D., a 60-year-old auto company executive, was in so much pain he thought it was ordinary foot trouble. His podiatrist prescribed different types of shoes but the "rocks" were there all the time in his feet.

He couldn't work in the garden, ride his bike, drive a car or go for walks with his wife. His condition kept him from being sociable. He feared a pain attack while walking down the street. He would stumble. The attacks recurred with more and more frequency until he feared becoming an invalid.

A pain specialist performed a thorough diagnosis. Bill D. had an excessive outpouring of pain-causing prostaglandins and a deficiency in his immune system to balance the inflammation-causing arachidonic acid. His specialist suggested boosting consumption of Omega-3 fatty acids via daily intake of different types of seafood as well as concentrated fish oil capsules.

Within three weeks, the stabbing pains subsided; his inflammation cooled. He could soon walk, work, ride, drive, and even jog with virtually no discomfort. For fun, he'd even go barefoot around the house and enjoy this new freedom from arthritis pain.

How Fish Oils Produced Healing

Bill D.'s agonizing pain was traced to an excessive production of inflammatory compounds. The fish oils contained rich concentrations of EPA and DHA which protected the body against attack by its own immune system. Omega-3 fatty acid EPA and DHA helped cool the leukotriene substances that created tender joints and inflammatory discomfort. By boosting consumption of seafood, almost on a daily basis, together with the fish oil capsules, he corrected the imbalance in his immune system and his body was relieved of the searing pain. His immune system was stabilized with the nutrients in fish oil.

TUNA IS SOURCE OF OMEGA-3 FATTY ACIDS

"Does water-packed tuna supply the same level of Omega-3 fatty acids as oil-packed tuna?"

Several universities were queried and came up with the answer that water-packed tuna probably gives you more Omega-3 fatty acids. Reason? The oil used in oil-packed tuna is primarily soybean oil, which does *not* provide any Omega-3 fatty acids.

Since Omega-3 fatty acids are fat-soluble, a certain amount leaches out into the vegetable oil. When you drain the oil from oil-packed tuna, 15 to 25 percent of the Omega-3 fatty acids is lost, but by discarding the water of water-packed tuna, only 3.1 percent is lost.

Both Penn State University and the Massachusetts Nutrition Resource Center went beyond the Omega-3 question to say that water-packed tuna also has an advantage in less calories and fat. The numbers: 100 grams (3.5 ounces) of drained oil-packed tuna deliver a chunky 8.2 grams of fat and 200 calories, while the water-packed variety swims by with only ½ gram of fat and 131 calories.[4]

OMEGA-3 FATTY ACIDS AND JOINT PAINS

Andrew William Sereda, M.D., Neurologist, of Edmonton, Alberta, Canada, tells us:

"The most common form is osteoarthritis, also known as wear-and-tear arthritis, which is thought to occur as a result of overuse of joints. It is most prominent in older persons and at times is assumed to be an accepted accompaniment of aging.

"I have come to the conclusion that many of the symptoms and signs of aging can be attributed to a state of chronic malnutrition, especially with regard to a deficiency of antioxidant factors and excess intake of rancid fat and a breakdown in the immune system."

Dr. Sereda comments on the popularity of cod liver oil that was once said to be taken on an empty stomach, in an emulsified or mycelized form by shaking with orange juice:

---

[4] *Prevention Magazine,* May, 1988, pp. 35–38.

"We now have some idea of the importance of the anti-oxidant properties of Vitamin A, the calcium-mobilizing properties of Vitamin D, and the complex and tremendously important functions and interactions of the highly unsaturated Omega-3 fatty acids found in fish oil, including eicosapentaenoic acid (EPA) and docosahexaenoic acid (DHA).

"Even though these ideas about how cod liver oil lubricates the joints may seem quaint in contrast to other complex theories as to how it might work, they may eventually be proven to be partly right in this regard.

"Nonetheless many people have tried this method and have greatly benefited regardless of how or why such apparent spontaneous remissions occurred. If this is a placebo effect or wishful thinking, what difference does it make to the patient who benefited from the treatment program?

"With current knowledge of the importance of fish-oil-derived fatty acids in the prevention and treatment of atherosclerotic vascular disease (enhanced by other important dietary factors), the overall benefits seem to vastly outweigh any objections to its use."[5]

CRIPPLING PAINS WASHED AWAY WITH FISH OILS

Alice C. was troubled with multiple joint involvement from her arthritis. At times, her hips and knees were so pained she could only lie on her side; it was difficult to sit in a hard-backed chair. Medications created so many side effects, she would rather endure the arthritis as the "lesser of both evils." Was she destined to become an invalid?

A rheumatologist felt that a "whole patient" approach was indicated. She was given fresh foods, anti-oxidant vitamins, and increased amounts of seafood. She was also given fish oil capsules as well as cod liver oil on a daily basis.

The Omega-3 fatty acids caused a diminution in spasms, correction of prostaglandin synthesis. The EPA and DHA sub-

---

[5] *New Concepts in Prevention and Treatment of Nervous System Symptoms and Illnesses,* Andrew William Sereda, M.D., Edmonton, Alberta, Canada, 1987.

stances acted as mediators to guard against pain-causing leukotriene overload and threatening arachidonic acid.

Alice C. was soon able to experience a reduction of pain and swelling so that she could turn over in bed without crying out for help; she could sit in a wooden chair with no discomfort. Four weeks later she could not only move with youthful flexibility, but could ride a bicycle and participate in a local jogging race with agility and vitality. Her crippling pains were literally "washed away" because of the EPA-DHA balance of her prostaglandins and restoration of a stronger immune system.

FISH OILS BOOST IMMUNE SYSTEM

Omega-3 is a polyunsaturated fatty acid that occurs predominantly in deep-sea saltwater fish. It is similar, but not identical to Omega-6, the polyunsaturated oil found in vegetables. One of the major dissimilarities between these two fatty acids is an apparent interference in the way platelets—the coagulating components in the blood—stick together when Omega-3 is present. With these fish oils, blood platelets tend to be less sticky and less able to stick together or to blood vessels. In essence, the blood is thinned and flows more freely.

It is this thinner blood that is believed to be a key to a healthier metabolism and a stronger immune system to resist arthritis. Fish oil decreases a substance or antigen suspected as an invader in the immune system that could trigger arthritis inflammation. It makes good sense to have enough Omega-3 in your system for a stronger arthritis-fighting immune system.

IN REVIEW

1. An immune symptom of malfunctioning prostaglandins is often the cause of arthritis hurt and inflammation.
2. Scientists gave the name Omega-3 to certain polyunsaturated fatty acids to describe their molecular structure. These fatty acids strengthen the immune system and regulate prostaglandin balance to ease and overcome arthritic symptoms.
3. Fish oils buffer the painful inflammation-causing leukotrienes.
4. In medical trials, fish oils have been able to ease symptoms, correct inflammation, and strengthen tender joints.

5. Bill D. eased agonizing pains that made him feel as if he were walking on rocks with the help of immune-rebuilding fish oils.

6. Tasty seafood is rich in the EPA and DHA immune-strengthening substances to overcome arthritis. Tuna is another good source.

7. A folk remedy using cod liver oil may have scientific basis as a means of strengthening the immune system to cast out arthritis.

8. Alice C. was saved from crippling with the use of fish oils.

11

The Low Fat Way
to Free Yourself from
the Grip of Arthritis

Is fat clogging your arteries and cells? Has your immune system become sluggish because of a cholesterol overload? Have you weakened your immune system with excessive fat blockages? With a fatty barrier surrounding your cells, the defense system is unable to resist the onslaught of viral infections that could set the stage for arthritic disorders. Fat and cholesterol have been lumped together as "villains" to break down your immune response and open the floodgates to admit arthritic invaders.

BEWARE: FAT MENACE THREATENS
ARTHRITIS INFECTION

In order to appreciate the role that nutrition plays in the immune-building treatment of arthritis, it is helpful to become familiar with the basic metabolic procedure.

Arthritis: Immune Weakness

Arthritis is a weakness of the immune system of your body. Simply stated, this immune system protects you from invasion by germs, bacteria, viruses, and other agents that can do harm to your body. Fat and cholesterol are dangerous threats to your immune system.

The body's defense system consists of two components:

(1) *Alarm mechanism*—Identifies outside fat-cholesterol invaders in your body—similar to an alarm wired to the windows, doors, and trunk of an auto. This immune response signal is initiated by white blood cells or the "T"-lymphocytes—*thinking* lymphocytes. They identify the fatty invaders in your joint spaces and sound an alarm. The objective is to try and get the excess fat-cholesterol removed to protect the immune system.

(2) *Battle mechanism*—Hears the alarm and leaps into protective action. Other white blood cells or "B"-lymphocytes—*battle* lymphocytes—gather together and plan to help wash out the fat-cholesterol enemies in your joint area. They do this by recruiting mediators of inflammation; that is, an interactive relay system of cells, molecules, and other substances needed to sweep out debris and fatty deposits from the body. The goal is to help free your body from the fatty invaders.

FAT VS. IMMUNE SYSTEM

Fatty plaques composed of cholesterol and other deposits accumulate on the inside wall of arteries and restrict the passage of blood. If the accumulation of plaques goes unchecked, it restricts the blood flow that carries oxygen and vital immune-boosting nutrients to the tissues and organs. A buildup of fatty deposits clog the arteries, cells, and molecules and weaken the defense system. The "T" and "B"-lymphocytes cannot sound the alarm system, and viral invaders sweep within the body to predispose to arthritic conditions. Fat is the enemy of the immune system!

CHOLESTEROL AND FATS: GETTING TO THE ROOT OF THE PROBLEM

There is clear evidence that a large reduction in blood cholesterol and fats will stimulate the immune response to uproot and cast out arthritis-causing invaders. Who is in control of body accumulation of these dangerous enemies? You are . . . through your food intake. Some basic findings—

Cholesterol: An important fat-like substance found in every living body cell. It is a building block of the outer membrane of cells; an important component of the fatty sheath that insulates nerve fibers. Also required for production of digestive juices, Vitamin D, and sex hormones such as estrogen. The liver produces about 80% of your body's cholesterol; the rest comes from foods you eat. *Note:* Cholesterol is found only in foods of animal origin; there is none in fruits, vegetables, or grains.

Triglycerides: Lesser known but an overload is a threat to your immune system. A type of blood fat attached to a molecule of glycerol in the blood. Triglycerides are needed to provide your body's major source of energy from fat; they are the body's source of energy. A high or excess accumulation of these triglycerides can pose an immune risk by clogging cells and blocking the defense cleansers or the "T"- and "B"-lymphocytes. Your body becomes at high risk for arthritis invaders.

Excess cholesterol and triglycerides may accumulate in fatty streaks, form fibrous plaque, thicken the artery wall, and hamper normal blood flow. Your body becomes vulnerable to arthritis invaders.

KNOW YOUR CHOLESTEROL LEVEL

It is important to know your cholesterol level in order to boost your immune system to resist arthritis. A simple blood test determines your cholesterol level and is available through your health practitioner. The guidelines below will help you when discussing your cholesterol level and its effect on your immune system:

BLOOD CHOLESTEROL LEVEL GUIDELINES		
Age	**Moderate Health Risk**	**High Health Risk**
2–19 years	Greater than 150	Greater than 185
20–29 years	Greater than 200	Greater than 220
30–39 years	Greater than 220	Greater than 240
40 years +	Greater than 240	Greater than 260

Source: Blood Cholesterol-Consensus Conference, *Journal of the American Medical Association,* April 12, 1984—Vol. 253, No. 14.

While it is important to know your total blood cholesterol level, a more accurate index of immune risk is your level of two substances known as:

High-density lipoprotein—A "good" molecule that carries cholesterol out of the bloodstream, cleanses cells-tissues, and helps create a stronger immune system.

Low-density lipoprotein—A "bad" molecule that accumulates cholesterol and deposits it upon blood vessels and other tissues to inhibit and resist immune defenders.

Your Goal: More HDL and less LDL for a stronger immune system. *Example:* Desirable HDL is over 35; desirable LDL is under 130.

Your desirable blood cholesterol reading should be under 200.

Levels of fat and cholesterol in the blood at any given time are determined by body chemistry and diet (Figures 11–1 and 11–2.) With the following basic guidelines, you are in control of the storage of these immune system components.

First Line of Defense: Plan a meal program low in cholesterol (found in eggs, meat, poultry, seafood, dairy products) and saturated fats (animal fats and vegetable oils such as palm and coconut oil). Immunologists recommend the following:

1. *Reduce cholesterol intake* to less than 300 milligrams a day.

2. *Reduce total fat intake* to less than 30% of total calories.

3. *Restrict saturated fat intake* to less than 10% of total calories. Allow up to 10% of total calories from polyunsaturated fats. Allow 10% to 15% of total calories from monounsaturated fat.

NOTE: If this does not lower high cholesterol, reduce saturated fats to less than 7% of total calories; cholesterol to less than 200 milligrams daily.

CAUTION: Labels on food products should be read carefully. Commercially processed foods are rich in eggs and egg solids and in saturated and hydrogenated (also saturated) fats.

Watching Your Cholesterol? Then Watch Your Use of These Foods:
(high in saturated fat and/or cholesterol)

Dairy Products

whole milk	evaporated/condensed milk
light/heavy cream	sour cream
ice cream	non-dairy creamers
whipped toppings	cheeses (most)

Protein Foods

"hamburger"	shrimp
fatty meats	organ meats
poultry skin	hot dogs
duck, goose	spare ribs
bacon, sausage	egg yolk
cold cuts	

Bread and Cereal Group

commercial: biscuits, waffles, cornbread, pancakes, muffins, egg or cheese bread	butter rolls snack crackers egg noodles

Fruits and Vegetables

avocado and any buttered, creamed, or fried fruit or vegetable unless with an acceptable fat

Fat and Oil

shortening, coconut or palm oil, partially hardened or hydrogenated vegetable oils, butter, lard, salt pork, bacon, meat drippings, gravies, and cream sauces, unless modified

Figure 11–1

HOW TO IDENTIFY THREE BASIC DIETARY FATS AT A GLANCE

1. *Saturated Fats:* Butter, milk, meat fat, palm and coconut oil, hard margarine, and shortening. *Immune Response:* Raises blood cholesterol.

2. *Polyunsaturated Fats:* Vegetable oils such as safflower, wheat germ, corn, and soybean; also in seafood. *Immune Response:* Lowers blood cholesterol.

3. *Monounsaturated Fats:* Olive, peanut, and avocado oils. *Immune Response:* Lowers blood cholesterol.

With controlled fat consumption, a lowering of cholesterol and overall obesity, the immune system is free to dispatch the vital lymphocytes that will "defuse" and "destroy" hurtful invaders that trigger arthritis infection.

ARTHRITIS "SURRENDERS" TO NUTRITIONAL IMMUNE PROGRAM

An early injury created a traumatic assault that eventually opened the way to a viral infection with arthritis symptoms for Jessica MacC. She developed stiffness of her joints. As a computer programmer, she had recurring painful spasms in her fingers and wrists. At times, shooting pains down her spine made her wince with agony as her lower back became stiff with a crippling-like immobility. Was she going to surrender to increasing arthritis?

An immunologist diagnosed Jessica MacC.'s very high cholesterol-fat levels. He explained that her immune system could gather disease-fighting molecules but they could not penetrate her cells and joints because of the cholesterol-fat blockages:

"Your body is at war—arthritis invaders versus immune defenders. We'll use a diet approach to repel and drive out arthritis enemies. Once your arteries and cells are reasonably free of the obstacles formed by fatty cholesterol, your immune system is then able to help create an inner cleansing and restoration of health. You will have a stronger immune system to repel infectious invaders and resist arthritis among other ailments."

A reduction in animal-saturated fatty foods together with restriction of excessive calories soon reduced her obesity. Tests showed her cholesterol-triglyceride levels were being lowered. *Meaning:* Infectious invaders were overcome. Within five weeks, her flexibility was restored. Her hands could work swiftly on

Cholesterol and Saturated Fat Content of Various Foods

	Portion Size	Cholesterol (mg)	Saturated Fat (g)	Saturated Fat Calories
Fats and oils				
Butter	1 tbsp	31	7	63
Lard	1 tbsp	12	5	45
Shortening				
Animal and vegetable	1 tbsp	7	5	45
Vegetable	1 tbsp	0	3	27
Tallow (beef fat), edible	1 tbsp	14	6	54
Margarine				
Corn oil (stick)	1 tbsp	0	2	18
Soybean	1 tbsp	0	2	18
Corn oil (tub)	1 tbsp	0	2	18
Soybean oil (tub)	1 tbsp	0	2	18
Margarine, diet	1 tbsp	0	1	9
Oils				
Coconut	1 tbsp	0	12	108
Corn	1 tbsp	0	2	18
Olive	1 tbsp	0	2	18
Palm	1 tbsp	0	7	63
Palm kernel	1 tbsp	0	11	99
Peanut	1 tbsp	0	2	18
Safflower	1 tbsp	0	1	9
Soybean (partially hydrogenated)	1 tbsp	0	2	18
Sunflower	1 tbsp	0	1	9
Related products				
Mayonnaise	1 tbsp	8	2	18
Peanut butter	1 tbsp	0	2	18
Dairy products				
American cheese	1 oz	27	6	54
Cheddar cheese	1 oz	30	6	54
Cottage cheese				
Creamed, 4% fat	1 cup	34	6	54
Low-fat, 1% fat	1 cup	10	2	18
Cream	1 oz	31	6	54
Mozzarella (made with part skim)	1 oz	16	3	27
Parmesan, grated	1 tbsp	4	1	9
Swiss	1 oz	26	5	45
Cream—Half and Half™	1 tbsp	10	2	18
Cream, sour	1 tbsp	5	2	18
Cream products				
Imitation (contains coconut or palm kernel)	1/2 fl oz	0	1	9
Milk				
Whole, 3.3% fat	1 cup	33	5	45
Low-fat, 2% fat	1 cup	18	3	27
Low-fat, 1% fat	1 cup	10	2	18
Nonfat skim	1 cup	5	0.4	4
Buttermilk, cultured	1 cup	9	1	9
Milk dessert, frozen				
Regular ice cream, 10% fat	1 cup	59	9	81
Ice milk				
Soft serve, 2.6% fat	1 cup	13	3	27
Sherbet, 2% fat	1 cup	14	2	18
Yogurt				
Made with low-fat milk	1 cup	11	2	18

Figure 11–2

Cholesterol and Saturated Fat Content of Various Foods (cont'd)

	Portion Size	Cholesterol (mg)	Saturated Fat (g)	Saturated Fat Calorie
Fish, shellfish, meat, and poultry (cooked)				
Beef				
Chuck arm pot roast, cooked lean	3 oz	85	3	27
Chuck blade, lean	3 oz	90	5	45
Flank, lean	3 oz	60	5	45
Rib (6-12)	3 oz	69	5	45
Rib eye (10-12)	3 oz	68	4	36
Rib (6-9)	3 oz	70	5	45
Round, full	3 oz	70	2	18
Round, bottom	3 oz	81	3	27
Round, eye	3 oz	59	2	18
Round tip, lean	3 oz	69	2	18
Round top, lean	3 oz	72	2	18
Tenderloin, lean	3 oz	72	3	27
Top loin	3 oz	65	3	27
Sirloin	3 oz	76	3	27
Ground beef, 15% fat	3 oz	70	5	45
Ground beef, 20% fat	3 oz	74	7	63
Pork				
Center rib roast chop				
Lean and fat	3 oz	69	7	63
Lean only	3 oz	67	4	36
Sirloin roast	3 oz	83	4	36
Canadian bacon	2 slices	27	1	9
Spareribs, lean and fat	2 slices	103	10	90
Cured bacon	3 slices	16	3	27
Veal cutlets	3 oz	86	4	36
Lamb loin chop, lean only	3 oz	80	4	36
Poultry				
Dark meat without skin	3 oz	79	2	18
Light meat without skin	3 oz	72	1	9
Fish				
Flounder or sole, lean fish	3 oz	59	0.3	3
Salmon, red fatty fish	3 oz	60	1	9
Shellfish				
Shrimp	3 oz	134	0.2	2
Lobster, northern	3 oz	90	0.1	1
Oyster	3 oz	45	0.5	5
Related products				
Frankfurter, beef	1	27	7	63
Bologna, beef	1 slice	16	3	27
Salami	1 slice	18	2	18
Braunschweiger	1 slice	44	3	27
Egg yolk, large	1	274	2	18
Egg white, large	1	Trace	0	0
Baked goods				
Cake, frosted				
Devil's food, frosted	1/12 8″ layer	50	5	45
Yellow cake, frosted	1/12 8″ layer	36	3	27
Brownie with icing	1	13	2	18
Chocolate chip cookies	4 cookies	21	4	27
Doughnuts, cake	1	10	1	9
Doughnuts, yeast	1	13	3	27

Figure 11–2 (Cont'd.)

her computer. When she sat before her video display terminal, she felt agile and alert. Her back was mobile again. She could say "goodbye" to arthritis because it had "surrendered" to a boosting of her immune system. It was accomplished with a balanced cholesterol-triglyceride-fat level.

HOW TO FIGHT BACK AND WIN THE ARTHRITIS BATTLE

Your body may fall prey to the threat of arthritis via the entrance of bacteria, viruses, and other microorganisms. This does not have to be. Instead, you need to boost your natural defenses and powers of immunity against this arthritis-causing invasion.

Phagocytes, Neutrophils, Macrophages

Invigorate your immune system with powerful white blood cells and protein molecules that can effectively win against arthritis invaders. A low-cholesterol, low-fat program will reduce threat of fat-clogged tissues. "Clean" arteries and joints become more resistant to invaders. In particular, your immune system releases phagocytes (the name means "eater cells"), such as neutrophils, which are short-lived arthritis fighters designed for the big attack; also, macrophages ("big eaters") are slower cells which back up and then wipe out arthritis invaders missed by neutrophils, and which clean up the debris left after the battle.

These cells are your immune system's soldiers. They do combat with arthritis invaders, attaching to them, killing them with cleansing substances, and digesting them with proteins known as enzymes.

Break Down Resistant Arthritis Barriers

Easily done! To muster the outpouring of these arthritis fighters, simple dietary changes will help reduce fatty blockages and make it easier for your phagocytes to keep your limbs and joints free of hurtful microorganisms. Suggestions include:

*Eat less butter, margarine, and other fats overall; eat fewer fried foods.

*Substitute polyunsaturated oils for butter.

*Choose fish, poultry, and lean cuts of meat; either limit or entirely eliminate sausage, bacon, and processed luncheon meats.

*Trim fat from meats before cooking; remove skin from poultry before eating.

*Eat less organ meats such as liver, kidney, or sweetbreads.

*Use skim or low-fat dairy products such as cheese, milk, and yogurt; choose ice milk over ice cream.

*Eat more foods high in fiber such as fruits, vegetables, whole grains, and cereals to replace high-fat foods.

*Cut down on baked goods made with lard, coconut oil, palm oil, or shortening.

*Use fewer egg yolks and more egg whites in cooking.

*For salad dressings, reduce oil in half; substitute low-fat, plain yogurt.

*To sauté foods, try a non-stick pan. Use a small amount of salt-free vegetable stock in place of any fat; if necessary, apply a thin coat of oil with a pastry brush.

*Instead of coating fish with butter, wrap in a lettuce leaf before baking to retain moisture. Remove lettuce before serving.

*Try this healthful substitute for fatty mayonnaise or sour cream: Combine two-thirds low-fat cottage cheese with one-third low-fat, plain yogurt in blender or food processor.

*Thicken sauces with a vegetable purée. A good thickener is a mashed or puréed potato.

*Sweeten dishes without sugar by using concentrated fruit juices such as frozen orange or apple juice.

*Enjoy a smooth, creamy custard or flan by using evaporated skim milk instead of whole cream or milk. Substitute egg whites for whole eggs when making these desserts.

*For egg recipes, substitute egg white for yolk in the following ratios—one egg white for one egg yolk, two egg whites for one whole egg, and three egg whites for two whole eggs.

*Egg yolks are very high in cholesterol. One yolk has about 274 milligrams, almost your total daily limit. You may try a commercially prepared product which has the yolks removed. It consists of egg whites artificially cooked and flavored. When cooked, it is almost identical to scrambled eggs in taste, texture, and appearance.

By making these simple changes, you help cleanse your body of accumulated or excess cholesterol. In so doing, you enable your body to send forth strong immune forces to do battle with arthritis invaders and achieve victory, thanks to less fatty barriers!

OAT BRAN: POWERFUL FAT-BUSTING, IMMUNE-BUILDING FOOD

Oat bran may be the most powerful weapon available for the immune system to chase out arthritis invaders without the interference of cholesterol.

Secret Power of Oat Bran

It is a richly concentrated source of soluble fiber and blood glucans which create a viscous property to help attach to cholesterol invaders and wash them out of the system. Oat bran has a cleansing reaction on lipid and glucose metabolism to help speedily lower cholesterol. It is one of the few fibers that helps keep cells and tissues and arteries cleansed so that the immune defense system is successfully able to defuse and destroy arthritic invaders.

Oat bran is also high in protein. Its PER (Protein Efficiency Ratio) is higher than other grains to provide greater force to the phagocytes, neutrophils, and macrophages to wipe out arthritis invaders.

HDL-LDL Ratio Kept in Fighting Shape

It is one of the few foods that will *raise* important immune-boosting HDL levels and *lower* virus infectious LDL levels. Other foods may reduce levels of *both* lipoproteins and this could create an unhealthy balance. Oat bran maintains strong HDL levels to keep your arthritis-fighting phagocytes in top form.

When oat bran is used with a low fat meal program, your immune system becomes stronger because of eliminated infectious invaders.

HOW TO USE SOLUBLE FIBER FOR EASY CHOLESTEROL CONTROL

Basically, it is found in oats (also in dried beans, apples, oranges, and barley, although to a smaller degree) and can be enjoyed in many ways:

*Substitute oat bran for up to one-third of the flour in baked goods or as breading for oven-fried seafood.

*Add 2 tablespoons of regular or quick-cooking rolled oats to 2 cups of brown rice and use as a side dish.

*Toast rolled oats with a bit of oil and cinnamon in a 350°F. oven. Serve as a topping for low-fat yogurt or cottage cheese.

*Use ⅓ cup of oats instead of bread crumbs for any fish or vegetable or meat loaf for every 1 pound of the filling.

*About 50 grams of oat bran a day—the amount in a typical serving of oat bran hot cereal—will give your body the needed power to eliminate undesirable low-density lipoproteins and boost the effectiveness of a free-moving immune response to deal with arthritis invaders among other infections.

UPROOTS, CASTS OUT ARTHRITIS ON AMAZING FIBER PLAN

Being overweight was only part of the problem faced by seed merchant Richard R. Y. He had a high fat-cholesterol reading. He felt increasing stiffness so that it was difficult for him to drive his station wagon from farm to farm and sell his seeds and agricultural supplies. His reflexes became slowed by a "tightness" in his shoulders.

At times, Richard R. Y. felt he had "painful knots" between his shoulders so that turning the wheel or moving his upper body became a dangerously slow process. His arthritis was worsening until he feared becoming immobile or chair-bound.

A rheumatologist believed in treating the "whole person" to get to the cause of the condition. He found that Richard R. Y. had unnaturally high levels of fat and cholesterol along with his overweight, and further tests showed a blockage of disease-fighting phagocytes.

He told Richard R. Y. that his immune system was "outnumbered" because of the fat-cholesterol blockages. The program called for a dietary change with low fat-cholesterol foods. He was also told to eat at least one or two oat bran muffins a day—or at least a bowl of oat bran cereal with apple slices in skim milk. With the backup of a nutritionally sound, calorie-controlled program, he soon lost much weight along with his excessively high cholesterol readings. At the end of six weeks, Richard R. Y. noticed his "shoulder knots" starting to become "untied." When he drove to sell his agricultural wares to different farms, he had greater flexibility at the wheel and in daily activities. Shortly thereafter, his arthritis was "uprooted and cast out," according to his rheumatologist.

Thanks to an invigorated immune system, the phagocytes could move freely to attack and devour and cast out the arthritis invaders and hurtful microorganisms. Richard R. Y. was saved from arthritis crippling with the cholesterol-scrubbing fiber plan that gave him a more-powerful, biologically boosted immune system!

HOW TO "OIL" YOUR JOINTS AND BECOME IMMUNE TO ARTHRITIS

Immunological scientists have discovered a vital connection between immunity to arthritis and the power of monounsaturated fatty acids found in olive oil.

To understand how olive oil is "food" for the immune army, here is a brief glance at important words and their meanings:

High-Density Lipoproteins (HDLs)—Carry cholesterol away from cells to be eliminated from the body and are known as "good" cholesterol.

Low-Density Lipoproteins (LDLs)—Deposit cholesterol in tissues, cause blockages to the immune-fighting phagocytes, and are known as "bad" cholesterol.

Monounsaturated Fats—Come from vegetable sources and contain one hydrogen atom less in their structure than saturated fats. They help reduce cholesterol levels in the blood and also may boost the levels of important HDLs . . . giving your immune system more "fighters" to combat arthritis-causing microorganisms.

IMMUNE-BUILDING POWER OF OLIVE OIL

New findings indicate that olive oil is able to keep constant the levels of HDLs while reducing the LDLs, thereby enabling your immune system to attack arthritis invaders without cholesterol blockages.

Olive oil, rich in monounsaturated fatty acids has the added advantage of *not* causing an increase in blood triglycerides which could otherwise cause further cellular blockages and interferences.

Which Olive Oil to Use?

The best quality is extra-virgin olive oil; it means simply that the oil contains no more than 1 percent of oleic acid. (The less oleic acid in the oil, the better the flavor.) Some connoisseurs say that the finest of extra-virgin oils are cold-pressed—meaning no hot water has been used to extract them—from the first pressing of the olives. Some extra-virgin oil is also available unfiltered, which gives it a greener, more olive-rich flavor than filtered oil.

Oils that are very low in acids are frequently blended with higher-acid oils to achieve the acid content of 1 percent or less. If you prefer the very finest extra-virgin oil, look for those that are unblended and clearly labeled "unfiltered, cold-pressed, extra-virgin olive oil."

In Brief: Extra-virgin means oleic acidity not exceeding 1 percent; super-fine virgin means acidity not exceeding 1.5 percent; fine virgin, not exceeding 3 percent; virgin, not exceeding 4 percent. It's largely a matter of taste.

Your health store has top quality products available. A rich tint and an emphatic bouquet and flavor will tell you the oil is tasty and healthful, too.

Clears Path for Immune Defenders

The problem begins when a high blood cholesterol level results in accumulation of fatty deposits in blood vessels throughout the body. This narrows the vessels, reducing blood flow and allowing a buildup of hard plaques that repel and resist immune defenders.

The solution would be in using olive oil because the monounsaturated fatty acids are synthesized speedily by the body, alert the immune system, and promote a cleansing of cell membranes. This clears the pathway for arthritis-fighting phagocytes.

(Olive oil contains 72.3 percent of monounsaturated fatty acids, making it a powerful ally of the immune system in cleansing hurtful arthritis-causing microorganisms.)

HOW A "CRIPPLED" ARTHRITIC BECAME "ATHLETIC" WITH OLIVE OIL

Office manager Amanda Z. felt increasing joint pain as the days and months wore on. Her fingers became so stiff at times, she could scarcely hold a pencil or make use of the office filing system. It was painful to grasp a handle and open a door or drawer.

She fervently hoped her arthritis would "go away" as she heard it did for others. While she experienced occasional spontaneous remission of symptoms, the arthritis returned with increased vengeance to make up for lost time! She feared being disabled. The inflammation as well as the hurtful spasms in her wrists, shoulders, and soon her hips and knees made her all the more worried. Would she become a wheelchair victim?

Her osteopathic physician used a total body approach. An examination showed she had unusually high levels of fat and cholesterol. Her immune system was weak, unable to penetrate the barrier of excessive and hostile pain-causing LDL microorganisms.

His program? A controlled-calorie-and-fat meal program with increased oat bran daily and little more than 2 or 3 tablespoons of olive oil daily. Exercise further helped to invigorate her sluggish immune system.

Results? In eight weeks, her weight was stabilized; perhaps more important, a blood test showed her HDLs were boosted while the harmful LDLs were lowered in a healthful ratio.

Amanda Z. was thrilled when finger-wrist-shoulder pains and stiffness "melted" away. It took a bit longer for her "oiled" immune system to fight off threatening arthritis viral invaders but by the end of the eleventh week, her hips and knees were mobile again. She no longer feared wheelchair crippling. Instead, she joined a tennis and jogging as well as swimming club and boasted how she would soon be an "athlete" with youthful flexibility. It was all due to the olive oil's invigorating effect on the HDLs to cleanse away plaque deposits so that the arthritis intruders were knocked out and eliminated!

HOW MUCH TOTAL FAT AND OLIVE OIL DAILY?

1. Based upon an estimate of total fat intake of less than 30 percent of daily caloric intake, you can aim for *15 to 18 teaspoons of fat per day.* This includes all fat: the unseen fat in foods such as meats and cheeses as well as the fat you see or put on foods.

2. Throughout the day, aim for no more than 2 or 3 tablespoons of olive oil—as part of the *total* amount of fat intake. That's all your immune system needs.

How to Stimulate the Immune System with Olive Oil

Some tasty suggestions include:

*When broiling or roasting meats or poultry, brush with olive oil to seal in natural juices. Adds a delicious flavor.

*Marinate meats and poultry in olive oil before cooking.

*Keep crispness and add flavor by popping corn in olive oil. Then drizzle olive oil over the top of the popped corn. Delicious!

*Add a teaspoon of olive oil to a serving of hearty soup.

*Marinate chicken in equal parts of olive oil and lemon juice before baking or broiling.

*Sauté fish fillets, sparked with tarragon and chives in olive oil.

*Dip eggplant, squash and potatoes in olive oil before baking—skins will stay firm and glossy.

*Season green vegetables with olive oil, lemon juice, and herbs.

*Toss your favorite pasta with olive oil, scallions, Parmesan cheese, and freshly ground pepper.

*The classic salad dressing is three parts olive oil to one part good wine vinegar—plus mustard and pepper to taste.

*Mash garlic cloves in olive oil and spread on crusty bread for grilling.

*A flourish of fruity olive oil with a squeeze of lemon juice is a favorite thrill for steamed vegetables.

*Take a tip from the "arthritis-free" Mediterraneans and add a dollop of olive oil instead of butter to a plate of steamed green vegetables—chard or broccoli—or over a gently poached fillet of white meat or fish.

Give your immune system a nutritional "shot in the arm" against invading arthritic microorganisms with the use of fat-cholesterol-fighting oat bran and olive oil. A low-fat and low-cholesterol meal plan will further invigorate your immune system to help uproot and cast out arthritis invaders!

IN REVIEW

1. Excessive fats, such as cholesterol-high foods, block the immune system and cause an arthritis risk if harmful microorganisms have taken hold.

2. A simple meal change with fewer saturated fatty and cholesterol foods helps keep joints free of hurtful bacteria that could trigger arthritis. See lists of "taboo" foods.

3. Help your immune system break down arthritis invaders with improved eating methods. Enjoy tasty suggestions.

4. Oat bran invigorates your immune system to cast out hurtful LDLs that might otherwise predispose to arthritis.

5. Jessica MacC. used a nutritional immune program to cause arthritis to "surrender."

6. Richard R. Y. cast out arthritis via an oat bran program that gave the majority power to his immune system.

7. Olive oil used by Amanda Z. helped create immunity to arthritis and eliminated the threat of becoming "crippled." She was athletic, instead, thanks to the power of a strengthened HDL ratio because of the olive oil.

12

The Immune-Stimulating Food That Heals Arthritis from Within

Boost the healing powers of your immune system with the use of garlic. Immunologists have found that common garlic is able to cause an outpouring of arthritis-fighting white blood cells and protein molecules to reverse the spread of this condition. This adds substance to the familiar folk tale that the small but mighty garlic bulbs can, indeed, fight the viral invaders of body tissues.

Garlic Boosts Immune System

Garlic reportedly so stimulates the immune system that it more than doubles the potency of natural healing cells, those powerful lymphocytes that eradicate arthritis-infected cells but leave normal cells unharmed.

ALLICIN: GARLIC'S THERAPEUTIC COMPONENT

Garlic has a wide range of detoxifying and anti-microbial benefits. These therapeutic properties are attributed to its many sulfur compounds; in particular, to allicin.

Power of Allicin

Allicin, or allyl allylthiosulfinate, is an active antibacterial ingredient found in garlic; it belongs to a family of compounds called thiosulfinates which function as bacteria and fungus-fighting agents. Allicin is created in garlic when an enzyme and amino acid combine to create a boosting action upon the immune system to "knock out" hurtful bacteria and virus invaders involved in arthritis disorders.

Garlic's allicin inhibits the growth of dangerous viruses through a reaction upon a group of sulfhydral substances in the body. Allicin has a bacteriostatic action; that is, it inhibits or blocks further growth of these arthritis-causing bacteria and creates a form of inner immunity against this infection. Allicin prevents the spread of infectious fungus invaders without upsetting the host organism. That is why you can eat garlic as a natural antibiotic without any side effects as would be the case with most drugs.

Garlic: Natural Antibiotic

As a member of the Liliaceae (lily) family, some of its relatives offer sulfur derivatives found in sulfonamides and penicillins. In tests, extracts of garlic have a powerful antibiotic effect. You can prove garlic's antiseptic potency by placing a crushed clove under glass, then setting next to it a culture or fungus. In a few minutes, all bacteria will perish.

A bacterial invasion is symptomatic of a weakness in the immune system that could lead to arthritis. This condition is not solely in one of the joints but frequently involves any tissue in the body. When harmful organisms spread, the same histological changes in the joint capsules may be found in extra-articular lesions and consist of inflammatory lymphocytic infiltration, formation of germinal follicles, and often plasmocytosis accompanied by arteritis, arteriolitis, or endarteritis. That is, inflammation together with extra-articular lesions. These are the so-called auto-immune infiltrations. They need to be checked, repelled, and cast out. It is garlic, through its natural antibiotic action, that is able to help reverse the tide of this bacterial invasion.

GARLIC, ARTHRITIS, IMMUNE SYSTEM

It has been reported by electrobiologists that garlic releases a strange type of ultraviolet mitogenetic emission. These emissions, referred to as Gurwitch rays, have the ability of nipping arthritis infection by stimulating cell growth and activity and strengthening the immune system.

The " virus-busting" power of garlic is found in its active factors: allistatin as well as germanium (trace mineral) which are useful against staphylococcus and escherishiacoli (E. coli), often found in arthritis conditions.

Garlic also boosts the immune system to help create an anti-oxidant reaction to cast out hurtful free radicals or enemy invaders that could trigger arthritis infection. Garlic helps to neutralize these toxins and strengthen the immune system to protect the body from harmful reactions.

GARLIC HELPS "COOL" INFLAMMATION

Inflammation is the cause of swelling, redness, heat, and pain of many kinds of arthritis. It is inflammation that leads to deformity and crippling. It is chronic and persistent.

Blame Inflammation on Virus Invasion

We usually relate viruses with acute illnesses such as flu or a bad cold. Yet viral invaders can also be responsible for arthritis inflammation. The virus invader penetrates the immune system, launches an attack, and causes body mechanisms to become abnormal in function. The result is joint inflammation or arthritis.

Garlic to the Rescue

Garlic, with its allicin substance, creates an anti-virus reaction which helps to "chase out" the harmful invader, strengthen the immune system, and create a natural cooling of inflammation. For arthritics who find the side effects of anti-inflammatory drugs worse than the condition, the use of garlic (it's a food!) may be a welcome alternative. Cooling, too!

SOOTHES ARTHRITIS IN EIGHT DAYS WITH GARLIC "MEDICINE"

Whenever John X. took a prescribed medicine promising to ease inflammation, he developed uncomfortable side effects. Dizziness caused problems on his assembly line job where his foreman scolded him for sleeping when he was unable to control a groggy feeling.

A change in medicine brought different side effects: constant thirst, eating disorders, gastrointestinal upset, and nervous spasms. John X. felt his job was in jeopardy because of his inability to concentrate or follow simple instructions from supervisors.

A co-worker told John X. of his own experiences with "hot" arthritis and how he relied upon an "old world" remedy to obtain relief. Garlic! Since he did not want to try other drugs because of the predictable discomforts, he decided to use garlic. A few cloves per day mixed in a raw vegetable salad was the suggested "remedy."

John X. felt minimal relief on the second day. He preferred "instant relief" and only upon the urging of his co-worker did he continue ingesting raw garlic. On the fourth day, his inflammation subsided somewhat, encouraging him to keep on the garlic program. By the seventh day, the hurtful heat was much, much cooler. He was so relieved on the eighth day, John X. called garlic his "natural medicine" and "arthritis healer." He was free of side effects and could work with speedy mental and physical efficiency, thanks to the immune-strengthening power of cooling garlic!

GARLIC HELPS "TURN ON" THE IMMUNE SYSTEM

Garlic is much more than an immune enhancer. It has the broadest spectrum of any anti-microbial substance that we know of—garlic is anti-bacterial, anti-fungal, anti-parasitic, anti-protozoan, and anti-viral. This gives garlic a powerful force that arthritis invaders have to contend with.

T-Cells Activated by Garlic

As an autoimmune condition, arthritis may be blocked by stimulation of the T-cells or defensive white blood cells. T-cells are required to "turn on" the immune system in all of its forms. Garlic acts as a stimulus; it prompts the immune defenses to produce antibodies that attack the invading agents. Garlic stimulates other T-cells to protect various infected body cells. Since arthritis is a "whole body" condition, the T-cells travel throughout the entire body to search for and ultimately "knock out" hurtful invaders.

It is garlic that calls the T-cells to order and dispatches them to different parts of the body. Garlic further stimulates antibody formation. Macrophages (scavenger or cleansing cells) ingest foreign substances such as the arthritis virus and eliminate them from the system.

The garlic-prompted T-cells come by, via the bloodstream. (Now you understand the importance of a cholesterol-controlled bloodstream and cleansed cells and tissues.) These T-cells "see" the viral fragments presented to them by the macrophages and—in a counterattack against the invader—activate the immune system to attack that particular virus wherever it is found.

Strengthening the Immune System

A foreign invader can be a virus, bacterium, or anything else that does not belong in the body and represents a threat. A healthy immune system hurries to defend the body against arthritis infection. It uses its defender blood cell called a lymphocyte.

Importance of Lymphocytes

These are a kind of protective force circulating throughout the body. They spot the enemy and then leap into action. The lymphocytes change into plasma cells which then manufacture antibodies that are specifically designed to destroy the arthritis-causing invaders. If the immune system is weak, these lymphocytes become sluggish and "loaf" on the job which allows arthritis infection to spread. To stimulate the production and activity of lymphocytes, the use of garlic has long been recognized as an immune stimulant.

HOW AND WHY GARLIC STIMULATES THE IMMUNE SYSTEM

Garlic (allium sativum) is richly endowed with a number of active factors that help boost the immune system. These include:

Allicin—Substance believed to have a valuable anti-bacterial and anti-inflammatory benefit.

Allinin—A sulfur-containing amino acid which has a valuable natural antibiotic effect.

Diallyldisulphide-oxide—A cholesterol and fat-washing factor that helps cleanse cells so the valuable lymphocytes can pass through easily to uproot and cast out harmful bacteria.

Gurwitch rays—A mitogenetic radiation factor that encourages cellular rejuvenation and helps stimulate all body functions, particularly the immune system.

Anti-oxidant reaction—Garlic inhibits peroxidation (rancidity) and is considered able to help create elimination of free radicals or unpaired molecules that often trigger arthritis pain.

Selenium—A little-known trace element that has anti-atherosclerotic reactions. It protects against clot formation and platelet adhesion. Garlic's selenium is also an anti-oxidant factor; its biological activity has an inhibiting action on the formation of hurtful free radicals.

For the arthritic or anyone else concerned about a strong immune system (who isn't?), garlic may well be a "magic bullet" in our modern times.

FROM "WHEELCHAIR ARTHRITIS" TO "JOGGING CHAMPION" IN SIX WEEKS

Worsening inflammation and near crippling joint stiffness made Ruth B. feel so helpless, not to mention frightened about the prospect of becoming an invalid, that she took to her wheelchair for fear of hurting herself further.

Medications provided some relief but she had such aching knees and legs, she was understandably cautious about walking or moving about without the help of her wheelchair or an occasional cane. If she used a "walker," she felt more like an invalid which brought on tears and self-pity. She was terrified of being institutionalized if her condition worsened.

Fortunately, a neighboring microbiologist suggested tests to determine if her immune system was as depressed as her emotions. Laboratory reports confirmed a sluggish T-cell situation.

Her body needed stimulation to alert these lymphocytes into action to uproot and cast out the viral invaders detected under the microscope as the reason for her arthritis.

Ruth B. was concerned about interactions of different drugs (some could be fatal!) so opted for a recommendation to try garlic. She consumed at least five or six large cloves daily along with a raw vegetable salad.

Within two weeks, the inflammation "just went away." In four weeks, the so-called crippled joints became "healed" and she had a "miraculous" restoration of flexibility. She was able to leave her wheelchair during the fifth week. No cane or "pitiful" walker, either. She needed more proof of her healing. She joined a jogging group with the approval of her health practitioner. At the end of the sixth week, she not only could jog daily but entered a contest and was proclaimed champion against others who were more experienced runners. "I didn't win," she boasted to the news media. "It was garlic that saved me from arthritis. Garlic is the champion!"

HOW TO USE GARLIC FOR A STRONGER IMMUNE SYSTEM

Enjoy this "miracle food" in a variety of ways. To begin—

*Select garlic heads that are fat, solid, and unsprouted. Some prefer them loose instead of boxed or prebagged in plastic.

*Store garlic in a dry, dark, cool place.

*If you need to store for several months, separate cloves, put in a small glass jar, cover with vegetable oil, use a screw type cap, and refrigerate. When down to the bottom, use the garlic oil as part of a salad dressing.

*Separate a garlic head into cloves by rapping on it with the heel of your hand. To peel: place clove on a cutting surface and rest the flat side of a heavy knife over the bud. Wrap smartly on the knife with your fist. The skin peels off easily.

*Mince garlic easily by adding some onion powder to the cloves before chopping. This minimizes scattering garlic all over your counter top.

*Remove garlic aroma from your hands by rubbing them with a lemon. You could also rub your fingers on a washcloth under running water; then wash your hands with soap and water.

*Neutralize the anti-social garlic breath by simply chewing fresh celery or parsley or munching on a clove.

*For puréed garlic, mash in a mortar or on a board with the flat side of a knife.

*To remove garlic smell from your hands, rinse in cold water, then rub with tomato juice or salt, and finish with a soap-water wash.

*Raw garlic has a sharp sting; to minimize, toss a cut clove with salad greens (include parsley and celery).

*Garlic's characteristic sting may be eased without flavor loss if whole, unpeeled heads are simmered à la grecque— together with some olive oil, lemon juice, oregano, and pieces of carrots and string beans.

*Roasting unpeeled garlic cloves in a pan of some broth along with a main dish also has savory results.

*Frying or sautéeing should be done carefully; the smaller the bits of garlic, the more essential the timing. Garlic should *never* be allowed to take on any hint of blackness.

*Enhance a vinaigrette dressing by adding whole peeled garlic cloves to the oil, vinegar, and seasonings and letting the mixture sit overnight or longer. You have a mild garlicky dressing without little shards of acrid taste.

*Garlic diminishes in taste and smell when it's cooked so use less for a salad than for a cooked dish.

*In vegetable dishes that call for sautéeing in oil or butter, toss some minced garlic in the fat just before adding the vegetables.

*Vegetable casseroles can get added zip from fresh garlic, too. Scatter minced garlic over the vegetables before baking. The fragrance is tantalizing!

*Use baked garlic cloves to spread on hot French bread.

*Too timid to try garlic? Remember that the strongest flavor comes from fresh, uncooked garlic that has been puréed or chopped. Whole garlic clove or cloves that have been cut in large pieces are milder. For the mildest sweet and nutty flavor, cook garlic for a long time in roasts, stews, or soups.

*When a recipe calls for minced garlic, remember that a medium clove minced, yields about ⅛ teaspoon.

*Make garlic vinegar. Add two or three fresh garlic cloves to each pint of vinegar. Let stand two weeks before using. Do the same with oil to be used in cooking or salad making.

Revitalize your immune system with garlic. It is a potent way of knocking out harmful viruses that would otherwise penetrate your immune system to create havoc.

Three small cloves daily may be eaten with a vegetable salad. Include garlic during cooking and in other recipes to further boost your immunity against arthritic viruses and harmful bacteria.

Small and powerful—garlic is an effective virus-buster!

Just as a single dose of medicine has been seen able to change body metabolism to ease arthritis, it seems astute to recognize that one single garlic clove possesses immune-strengthening substances that may free you from the grip of arthritis.

Garlic may well be the most powerful weapon your immune system needs to initiate healing of arthritis from within!

IN REVIEW

1. Garlic is a powerhouse of therapeutic components that many consider to be as effective as medicine for arthritis relief. It's natural, too!

2. John X. was able to stem the tide of his threatening arthritis and enjoy freedom from drugs and side effects with garlic . . . in only eight days.

3. Garlic's secret is in its ability to "turn on" your immune system to repel and cast out arthritis invaders.

4. Ruth B. went from "wheelchair arthritis" to "jogging champion" when her immune system overcame and cleared her body of arthritis with the help of garlic.

5. Enjoy garlic on a daily basis in a variety of tasty ways. Many call it a "magic bullet" in the immune-building battle against arthritis.

13

How to Use "Mind Power" to Correct Your "Arthritis Personality"

You may be arthritis-prone because of your emotional attitude. Stress, tension, negative thinking, pressure, overwork, unhappiness, depression—all weaken your immune system and lower your resistance to arthritis invasion.

The way you think may well be related to your "arthritis personality." You can think yourself ill. You should be able to think yourself well!

ANGER, HOSTILITY, ARTHRITIS

People with arthritis are often full of inner turmoil, likely to be excessively conscientious, fearful of criticism, frequently depressed, and have a poor self-image, says Robert Fathman, Ph.D., a Dublin, Ohio, Clinical Psychologist.

Dr. Fathman and Norman Rothermich, M.D., Professor Emeritus, Ohio State University, Columbus, conducted a study that evaluates the personality traits of rheumatoid arthritis sufferers.

Arthritis Personality Unmasked

"We found they have a personality that leads them to try overly hard to be nice to other people, to not lean on others for emotional support, and to stow things away down inside, especially anger," says Dr. Fathman. "They were remarkably conforming to these traits, which seem to precede the disease, not result from it."

Tension, Anger Problems

Many rheumatoid arthritis sufferers also had a situation of long-term tension or anger in their lives, Dr. Fathman adds. But these are people who will say everything's just fine when that couldn't be further from the truth.

Dominant Husband Causes Distress

"One woman first said that her husband was marvelous," Dr. Fathman recalls. "And as I started questioning her further, tears came to her eyes. It turned out that before they would go out in the evening, she had to stand inspection. Her husband would take a brush and do something to her hair, or tell her what she needed to do better for herself before they went out. Her husband was very controlling. She permitted him to be that way."

Triggers Arthritis

The end result, Dr. Fathman says, is that these people have so much repressed anger that it "eats them up." "The anger gets turned against the person's own self," Dr. Fathman comments. And in this case it might do so literally. Rheumatoid arthritis is thought to be an autoimmune disease, in which the immune system mutinies against the body.

PHYSIOLOGICAL-PSYCHOLOGICAL LINK

California psychiatrist George Solomon, M.D., and Rudolf H. Moos, Ph.D., both formerly at the Stanford University School of Medicine, discovered that people who are genetically predisposed to arthritis but are emotionally healthy avert the condition.

Blood Factor Examined

Drs. Solomon and Moos studied the blood factor found in most rheumatoid arthritis sufferers—and in about 20 percent of their healthy relatives. This "rheumatoid factor," as it is called, is an autoantibody—an antibody which, through some quirk of the immune system, reacts against the body's own protective antibodies.

Why Are Some Immune to Arthritis?

The question is raised: Why do some perfectly healthy people avoid arthritis despite this "genetic time bomb," the menacing autoantibody in their blood?

"The answer," say Drs. Solomon and Moos, "lies in their psychological profile. Physically healthy relatives of arthritis sufferers who tested positive for the rheumatoid factor were, *without exception,* emotionally healthy!"

By comparison, those relatives who were free of the autoantibody, represented a psychological cross-section of the general population—ranging from emotionally healthy to significantly disturbed.

Emotional Connection

Dr. Solomon comments, "We assume from this that if you have the rheumatoid factor in your blood but stay in good condition psychologically, you won't get arthritis. On the other hand, if you're genetically predisposed, and endure long periods of anxiety and/or depression or suffer some major emotional upset, you are at a high risk for arthritis."[1]

STRESS AND ARTHRITIS

John Baum, M.D., at the University of Rochester, examined the medical records of 88 children who were being treated for juvenile rheumatoid arthritis at a Rochester hospital. He tells

---

[1] *Archives of General Psychiatry,* "Emotions, Immunity, and Disease," 1964.

us that 28 percent of them came from broken homes. For half of these, the divorce or death of a parent had taken place within two years of the onset of the condition.

"Quite possibly, stress is a trigger for juvenile arthritis. It probably does not cause it, but it may set it off."[2]

Emotional Triggers

Emotional stress can trigger rheumatoid arthritis in a vulnerable person, "and once the disease has established itself, stress can make it worse," says George Ehrlich, M.D., Director of the Division of Rheumatology at the Hahnemann Medical School and Hospital in Philadelphia.

"Acute stress—losing your job, a death in the family, a divorce—can make arthritis flare up. It makes you vulnerable. When you're under stress, your body's defenses can be breached." Small, constant irritations are less dramatic but can be just as harmful.

"There is such a thing as wholesome stress," says Dr. Ehrlich. "A challenging job, for instance—that's exercise for the mind. It's unwholesome stress, frustration, that lays you open to the disease."[3]

Women and Arthritis

Dr. Robert Fathman comments, "There are social implications as well. Women have rheumatoid arthritis up to four times more frequently than men. I think it's because of what we do to little girls in our society. We teach them that it's wrong to get angry."

He suggests the use of supervised assertiveness training, relaxation techniques, and traditional group therapy. It has helped his rheumatoid arthritis patients function better. "They reported feeling less pain and were able to function better. They could identify stress with intensification of their pain very clearly."

Emotional factors often precipitate or contribute to the exacerbation of arthritis through a weakening of the immune system. An overload of stress upsets body balance and control.

---

[2] Press release, 1986.
[3] Press release, 1986.

Hidden anger also erodes the immune system, causes muscle tension, the invasion of hurtful bacteria, and the onset of arthritis.

WHICH STRESSES HURT THE IMMUNE SYSTEM

A psychiatrist and an arthritis specialist working together in London's Westminster Hospital found that almost all the women patients they treated reported a new stress just before the onset of their arthritic symptoms.

Specific Immune-Hurting Situations: A husband's firm went bankrupt; a woman had to move to an unpleasant job; a love relationship came to an end; a job folded up; a live-in lover moved in with another woman; a deeply distressed mother came to live with her daughter; an only child got married abroad; a close friend died.[4]

While these self-reports were after-the-fact, and therefore must be evaluated cautiously, these findings suggest that health practitioners treating arthritis should take into account recent events in patients' lives as well as the physical aspects of the condition.

YOUR ATTITUDE STRENGTHENS THE IMMUNE SYSTEM TO EASE ARTHRITIS

Be aware of your emotional state and any unusual stress which may be influencing your system. What determines the immune-hurting effects of stress is the extent to which your organism is pushed beyond your coping capacity. Your immune system weakens and your body becomes vulnerable to arthritis invaders.

Adjust Your Attitude

To protect against immune weakness, identify the events or conditions in your life that prove stressful. Understand how these affect the course of your arthritis. This initial step, in itself, relieves some of your stress and you may be able to

---

[4] *British Medical Journal,* June, 1981.

remove some of the stressors. Recognize stress . . . and then start to adjust your attitude to rebuild your immune system and shield yourself from arthritis flareup.

Identify Stress Symptoms

You can read your mind and body language to determine if you are being stressed. *Symptoms:* Cold hands, rapid breathing, rapid heartbeat, anxiety, forgetfulness, shakiness, headaches, muscle tension, knotted stomach. Your immune system is being threatened. Start to protect yourself.

TEN IMMUNE-STIMULATING, ARTHRITIS-HEALING HOME REMEDIES

1. *Be Aware of Changes.* Being subjected to several changes over a short period of time can cause such severe stress that you develop arthritis pain. Even minor changes can cause upset. Prepare in advance for change. Roll with the punches, not against them.

2. *Control Yourself in Crises.* You need not be alone. If facing any crisis, discuss things with friends or family. If necessary, seek professional help. Hidden within each crisis is an opportunity for change. Cope with the obstacles. Analyze the problem and list step-by-step methods for solution. Remain in charge of your feelings.

3. *Breathe Your Way to Relaxation.* Get in a comfortable position. To the count of ten, inhale slowly and deeply. Let your belly expand. As you exhale to the count of ten, visualize yourself breathing out stored-up tension. With each breath, tell yourself, "relax."

4. *Untie Those Emotional Knots.* Sit comfortably whether at a desk or on a chair. Inhale as you raise your arms and gently stretch them toward the ceiling. Wiggle your fingers for ten seconds. Now exhale while you let your arms go limp at your sides. Your attitude becomes relaxed as your mind becomes free of knots.

5. *Stretch Away Stress.* Still seated, stretch your legs out before you. Alternately flex and point your feet for ten seconds. Now point your feet and wiggle your toes for ten more seconds.

6. *Speak Up! You'll Feel Better.* Accumulated stress, whether thoughts or feelings, can store up immune-destroying tension. Become more assertive. Speak up! Express your feelings, whether sadness, joy, hurt, anger, or excitement. You'll feel better via a soothed attitude and a stronger immune system.

7. *Easing Stress While at Work.* If job pressures cause a feeling of panic or rush—*stop*—take a deep breath. Give yourself a few minutes to think things through. Instead of a coffee break, take a relaxation break. Stretch. Walk around. Do simple exercises. Shield your immune system from burnout by unwinding before you tackle new obligations.

8. *Think Your Way to a Stronger Immune Barrier.* Focus on a realistic and positive approach. Are you being unfair or unrealistic with yourself? CAUTION: These could be self-created traps: "I can't," "I must," or "If only" or "I wish." SUGGESTION: Give yourself "self-applause," or a pat on the back for any job well done. Did something fail? What did you learn from this experience? How has it been helpful? This positive approach eases stress and this protects your immune system to resist outside invaders.

9. *Soothing Ways to Relax.* Listen to soothing music. Exercise daily if only for 30 minutes. Try visualization such as imagery—picture a pastoral scene with all of your senses. What does it look like, smell like, taste like, sound like, feel like? Project yourself into that scene, mentally and physically. You will reprogram your mind to relax even under the most stressful of situations.

10. *Manage Time to Ease Stress.* At the start of each day, take a few moments to prepare a list of "things to do." Divide this list into "primary tasks," "secondary tasks," and "miscellaneous tasks." Continue until you have finished your list. *Careful:* Do not overschedule. Allow space for unexpected situations. *Important:* Reward yourself for tasks well done.

Emotional invigoration is a learned skill. There is a link between stress and the occurrence of arthritis because of a weakening of the immune system. These ten steps help "plug the gaps" in your immune system to resist infectious invaders.

"CASTS OUT" ARTHRITIS THROUGH
THOUGHT CONTROL

The sales supervisor was so jittery, she could hardly sit still when tabulating receipts at the start of the day. Lenore H. was troubled with arthritis flareups that would go into remission at times only to recur again. These sporadic outbreaks were diagnosed by her therapist as largely emotionally induced. Whenever Lenore H. faced deadlines, her wrists and shoulders experienced throbbing pain and nervous jitters.

Lenore H. was given a "mental prescription" based on the ten preceding immune-stimulating programs. She started to visualize comforting relaxation and the ability to handle chores on a step-by-step basis. One thing at a time. With prescribed breathing and stretching "stress-busters," she was able to protect against tightness and recurring aches while at work. By thinking her way to stronger self-control and more self-assuredness, Lenore H. stretched her immune system and was able to "cast out" hurtful arthritis symptoms.

Her jitters gave way to joy when her joints were freed of hurtful invaders and she had youthful flexibility once again.

THE MIND AND YOUR IMMUNE SYSTEM

A new science with a tongue-twisting name—*psychoneuroimmunology*—aims at defining the mind's effects on immunity and identifying the mechanisms by which it acts. Transient arthritic attacks triggered by the emotions are well-documented.

Personality, Coping, and Illness

Because the crucial factor seems to be *how* you cope with stressors, a number of studies measure what is variously called "hardiness," the "ability to cope," or "ego strength," and relate these to immune responses under stress. If you do not resist stress, you have fewer natural killer cells (responsible for defending against arthritis viruses) and could become victim to this condition.

Do You Have Emotional Hardiness?

It is a learned trait. You have it if you also have a sense of purpose in your work and life. You see challenges rather than threats. You feel in control. This hardiness will buffer life's events, decreasing their stressfulness and increasing immunity. If you are productive, you have emotional hardiness. If you are frustrated, you face danger of an immune breakdown.

FOUND: LINK BETWEEN BRAIN AND IMMUNE SYSTEM

The brain's hypothalamus (which governs the automatically operating nerves, most hormones, and links to emotions) is the likely source of messages to the immune system. Partial virus assault of the hypothalamus blocks immune responses. Immune cells are unable to feed messages back to the hypothalamus. One basic question is whether communication is by means of nerve signals, hormones, or both

Lymphocytes, the most vital arthritis-fighting immune cells, have receptors on their surfaces that bind a number of hormones and nerve cell chemicals including endorphins. These opiate-type brain cell products are possible messengers.

Whatever the messenger, it appears probable that the brain communicates directly with lymphocytes. Stress interferes and this causes disarray and a weakening of the immune system.

Cope with stress and you will be able to strengthen resistance against arthritis with a stronger immune system.

VISUALIZATION—VICTORY OVER ARTHRITIS WITH THOUGHT POWER

The newer science of psychoneuroimmunology recognizes that a technique called "visualization" or "guided imagery" is able to uproot and cast out hurtful arthritis-causing invaders. It musters the hypothalamus to send messages to the immune system to send forth important lymphocytes to stem the tide of the onrush of hurtful foreign invaders.

Easy Visualization Program: Sit in a comfortable chair or lie down in a quiet surrounding. No outside noises. Shaded lighting is restful. Visualize your arthritis invaders. Acknowledge that they are responsible for immune weakness and pain.

Visualize an outpouring of lymphocytes and phagocytes as being dispatched by your brain to strike and kill all hurtful invaders in their path. The lymphocytes zap the weaker parasites and then search out and annihilate all hurtful arthritis-causing bacteria.

Visualize a complete battle between your body's immune system against the arthritis enemy. Picture your lymphocytes and defensive white blood cells converging upon and consuming the dying or dead arthritis cells. Picture how your lymphocytes then carry the defeated enemy from the internal battleground to your liver and kidneys where the remnants of the once-threatening foe are flushed from your body forever.

Visualize a gradual strengthening of your immune system, a healing of hurt joints, tissues, and organisms. Envision freedom from arthritis because your "guided imagery" has won the battle!

How to Transform Imagination to Reality in Freedom from Arthritis

Picture your body's white blood cells preparing, then re-paving the surfaces of the joints of your arms or legs or wherever arthritis had taken hold. Imagine your lymphocytes carrying away all the debris of previous inflammations, patching any defects, giving yourself joints that are shiny, flexible, and slippery smooth. Visualize your healthy condition that you enjoyed before arthritis struck. Always envision arthritis as a weaker enemy and your lymphocytes as the stronger, victorious opponents, and you will help your brain send forth healing substances that will transform imagination to reality in the healing of arthritis.

WINS ARTHRITIS BATTLE WITH "MIND MOVIE"

Stephen I. faced a lifetime of drug-taking which did ease inflammation and hurtful spasms in his fingers and wrists. But side effects made him groggy, insomniac, and not in control of his thoughts. Recurring bouts of digestive upset and a suspicious rash that erupted after taking medicines made him concerned about his situation. Was the "cure" worse than the condition?

He attended a local seminar on the newer science of psycho-neuroimmunology and heard specialists tell of the importance of using "brain power" to send forth healing lymphocytes to overcome arthritis invaders that have penetrated the immune system.

He was told to try a "mind movie." That is, when in a quiet setting, visualize a motion picture screen. Stephen I. would write the script: unwelcome outsiders had entered his body. He would dispatch antibodies to battle these enemies. He could even use real people such as close friends, heroes, and heroines; role models; or Biblical persons such as David and Goliath. Obviously, David would be the good cells and Goliath would be the bad cells.

It was more than guided imagery. It was to be a full-length motion picture. In it, Stephen I. saw his uniformed lymphocytes charge into battle against the enemy virus organisms. He could even have a romantic involvement in which the leader of the good cells was in love with someone who was an arthritis victim. He had to zero in on the hurtful virus and destroy the enemy to save his loved one's life. It was a full-length film for as long as Stephen I. felt was adequate. In the end, the good cells won and the bad cells were destroyed and flushed out of the body.

It took four weeks before Stephen I. felt the "mind movie" was starting to heal his inflammation and pain. He conjured a series of such battles on a regular basis for variety. By the end of the seventh week, he could safely reduce his medication and hope for elimination of pain. His brain receptors had dispatched healing lymphocytes and he had visualized his arthritis out of his body. He enjoyed freedom from inflammation and such youthful flexibility of joints, he could play musical instruments with healthy enthusiasm. It was a smash hit movie! It won an award—for healing his arthritis!

TEN SPEEDY STRESS-BUSTERS TO BOOST THE IMMUNE SYSTEM

Unless you live in a vacuum, there's practically no way you can entirely remove stress from your life. You probably wouldn't want to, either. Life could be dull without the usual ups and downs, and it is boredom that, too, creates stress. The answer is to roll with the so-called punches. Recognize that stress has the ability to depress your immune system. This renders you vulnerable to invading viruses that predispose you to arthritis, among a host of other ailments.

Stress: Too Much Is Too Dangerous

Prolonged and unrelieved stress is a constant threat to your immune system. Decide you will have occasional periods of heavy-duty stress in your daily lifestyle. Your goal is to *minimize* the effects of stress. *Not* after undergoing long chemotherapy, but right now when stress is beating down on your immune system and opening the arthritis floodgates.

To help, here is a list of ten speedy stress-busters you can use right away. Find out what works best for you. Keep it available. Use the stress-buster(s) whenever you need to gain control over the event:

1. *Talk it out.* It's stressful to bottle up your concerns. Discuss problems with sympathetic ears. Write them out. Talk to yourself out loud if nobody is within reach. Get them out of your system and thereby ease the risk of weakening your immune barrier.

2. *Enjoy yourself.* It's easy to overlook this valuable stress-buster. When you have fun, you feel speedy relief from day-to-day tensions. Enjoy much laughter whether from books, films, games, or mixing with happy-go-lucky people. Laugh and your immune system becomes stronger. TIP: Try to anticipate when you are most vulnerable to stress. Plan recreation right after as a natural antidote. Laughter is a great medicine . . . without any dangerous side effects!

3. *Take a walk.* Casual walking, about 60 minutes at a clip, is a great form of recreation that helps ease neuromuscular tension. A brisk walk stimulates about 100 heartbeats per minute which promotes a balanced electrical muscular activity that will be soothing and comforting. When you feel stress mounting . . . take a walk!

4. *Massage is soothing.* You'll need help for this one. Remember how good it feels to have your back rubbed? (No

wonder cats purr.) You, too, will purr with a gentle rubdown. Either engage a professional massage therapist or else have your spouse or a close friend rub you where you feel tension pockets. (Return the favor because the kneading action upon another person is soothing to yourself.) During massage, the body's muscles, tendons, joints, skin, and fat tissues are alerted. Relief of muscle contractions (knots) helps you feel relaxed. You could also try a shower massage. There are specially fitted shower heads available at housewares dealers that force water out in soothing, rapid-fire pulsations on troubled spots. You can actually wash away your tension via a shower massage.

5. *Enjoy a warm bath.* Keep it comfortably warm. Extreme prolonged heat is too stressful. Bathwater at body temperature (98°) is a relaxing soak. Fill the tub, step in, sink down, place a rolled-up towel behind your head. Close your eyes. Visualize yourself on a tropical isle and let your imagination run free. You'll emerge a stronger person with a stimulated immune system.

6. *Adjust breathing rate.* When tense, ever notice how fast you're breathing? Shallow, too. Easy does it! Slowing your rate helps reverse the risks of overstress. Try slow breathing to a 7-second inhale and an 8-second exhale. Do four of those per minute for a total of 2 minutes and feel relaxed all over. You can do this stress-buster anywhere, anytime. No need to stop any other activity. It's an "instant" remedy for a stressful situation.

7. *Tell yourself to relax.* Ever-popular and successful meditation works wonders in helping to control heart rate, slow down breathing, and ease fluttery feelings. For a relaxation response, find a quiet setting. Select an object (word or sound), a passive attitude. Empty all thoughts and distractions from your mind. Make yourself comfortable. Close your eyes. Breathe slowly. Repeat the word or sound you've selected (like *one, health, vitality,* etc.) Every time you exhale, repeat the word. *Important:* Let your mind go blank. Do this up to 20 minutes. Many arthritics have found a sense of renewed well-being and refreshment because of this stress-buster. It tells you that your immune system is fighting back.

8. *Easy exercise boosts immunity.* Sit on the edge of a straight wooden chair, your knees about 12 inches apart, your

legs dangling forward at any angle greater than 90 degrees. Next—sit up very straight. Now let yourself collapse like a rag doll, your head forward, your spine rounded, your hands coming to rest on your knees. Then tell yourself: "My left arm is heavy, my left arm is heavy. . ." Repeat for 10 seconds while focusing thoughts on your arm from armpit to fingertips. Then make a fist. Flex your arms. Take a deep breath. Open your eyes. Repeat the procedure and go to your right arm. Then do the same for your left leg and your right leg. In this way, you relax your whole body from head to toe. All this in less than 15 minutes! A terrific immune-invigorator.

9. *Try a mind game to melt stress.* Your brain can be conned into doing what you suggest—sending forth virus-destroying lymphocytes—and melting stress while promoting the healing process. When stressed, you overreact your sympathetic nervous system. In a mind game, you calm down this system and ease reactions of your physiological being. Try this: When you are relaxed either in a chair or on a bed, focus upon a flower. Use *all* your senses. See the flower unfolding soft petals. Notice the color. Touch the flower. Feel the velvet texture. Enjoy the aromatic perfume of this beautiful flower. See more than one color. Perceive it. Experience it. Enjoy it! After five minutes, open your eyes. What was formerly tense or unbearable, now becomes easier to cope with. TIP: Let your mind "escape" to an exotic fantasy island, a happy childhood remembrance or whatever you enjoy. Search your psyche for what makes you happy and escape for only 5 minutes to return refreshed and stronger and much happier.

10. *The vitamin that boosts defenses.* To ease and erase much stress and boost your immune system, Vitamin C (ascorbic acid) comes to the rescue. It is a natural anti-stressor. When tense, your body produces an immune-hurting substance that lowers defenses. Vitamin C is said to detoxify that chemical and render it neutral. This vitamin is said to help produce a generous supply of adrenaline, a natural stimulant. Vitamin C helps your body release a moderate amount of adrenaline that helps resist the pressures of tense situations. It's found in citrus fruits.

You *can* overturn the odds in your favor. Arthritis healing is a natural function through stimulation of the immune system. Adjust your emotional attitude, cope with ups and downs . . . and with an arthritis-fighting immune system, you will come up—bursting with health!

IN REVIEW

1. Do you have an arthritis personality? With some simple adjustments in dealing with daily stresses, you can boost your immune system to help create healing with a happier personality.
2. Be alert to arthritis stress triggers and avoid or minimize their immune-threatening effects.
3. Use any or all of the ten immune-stimulating, arthritis-healing home remedies. They work swiftly.
4. Lenore H. happily "cast out" hurtful arthritis with thought control.
5. Visualization or "guided imagery" helps boost immune-building lymphocytes that also eject and destroy hurtful foreign invaders.
6. Stephen I. avoided being addicted to drugs by using a "mind movie" to create a powerful immune response to heal arthritis.
7. Try the ten speedy "stress-busters" anywhere, anytime to invigorate your immune system and defend yourself against arthritis.

14

Home Remedies That Quickly Erase Pain and Swelling

Many pain-troubled arthritics become caught up in a seemingly endless round of doctors' visits and hospital stays, searching for relief and fighting pain with bed rest, chemotherapy, and surgery—often to no avail.

With the newer knowledge of immunotherapy, the use of hydrotherapy, massage, and poultices, have been used to provide relief without the risk of side effects as is noted in drugs. Easily applied at home by yourself or a family member, these home remedies help provide relief by boosting your immune system to resist the mechanism of arthritis pain.

What Is Pain?

A physical signal, an alarm, signaling your body that something is wrong and attention is needed to prevent further injury. Local tissue injury or damage produces a pain message that is sent to the spinal cord, and then to the brain stem and higher segments of the brain where it is perceived as pain.

The Process of Pain

When a foreign invader has penetrated your weakened immune system, cells in the injured tissue release several substances (histamine, prostaglandin, and bradykinin) which stimulate local nerve endings and transmit pain messages toward the brain. Histamine attempts to fight off these invaders through an outpouring reaction; prostaglandin attracts blood cells to fight infection and in the process leads to swelling and inflammation; bradykinin is released to fight the invaders and causes a powerful pain during the defensive method. Your nerve endings are stimulated. They send an electrochemical impulse through the nerves to the spinal cord, through which nerve signals from all parts of the body must pass en route to the brain. From the spinal cord, the impulse moves up to the thalamus region of the brain and to the cerebral cord. Along the way, reactions occur. Spasms are sent via the pain pathways. Depending on how many nerve endings are involved in the arthritis, the pain can be mild, moderate, or severe.

How Pain Can Be Controlled

Your body has a "short circuit" mechanism by which pain can be quickly halted. Pain severity is specifically modulated by the release of *endorphins,* natural pain-killing chemicals found in the brain that inhibit the descending pain signals. To boost your immune response to pain, to "pull the plug" on these sensory impulses, you need to release more endorphins. You will then help your body ease and erase pain.

Simple Home Test to Ease Pain

Locate a part of your body subject to pain. For example, your shoulder. Now rub or press the painful area. It eases temporarily. *Reason:* Additional pressure overloads the pain pathway. More endorphins are released to "switch off" the hurt by blocking the painful bradykinin substance at the site of the hurt. It's as simple as that.

Pain Relief the Natural Way

To enjoy extended and long-lasting freedom from pain, you need to stimulate your immune system to block the painful bradykinin at the site of the injury. The use of simple home massage, hot and cold applications, simple water remedies help your immune system dispatch more endorphins to provide relief of pain the natural way.

HOW SELF-MASSAGE RUBS AWAY PAIN QUICKLY

Massage is a beneficial therapeutic home remedy for relaxation and revitalization of the mind and musculature. When you exercise or simply move about in daily activities, chemical byproducts (such as lactic acid) accumulate in your muscles. The metabolic byproducts are mostly eliminated and broken down by oxygen circulating through the bloodstream.

In a weakened immune system, residual byproducts remain in the tissue causing pain, fatigue, and that stiff, achy tightness you feel after strenuous exercise, moving and lifting, a day of yard work, or a day of simple housework.

Massage Acts as an Inner Cleanser

Massage works to speed up the removal of metabolic byproducts from the tissues by squeezing them out of the muscle fibers and back into the bloodstream for recirculation or elimination. Massage increases venous and lymphatic circulation. It stimulates blood flow which helps to nourish muscle tissue and increase joint mobility and flexibility. You will help send forth enough endorphins to counterattack the onrush of discomfort-causing histamine-prostaglandin-bradykinin invaders and cleanse your tissues and joints of hurtful irritants.

Use a Topical Rub

A lubricant is essential during self-massage because it reduces friction between the hands and the skin. It is helpful if you have sore muscles or joints. It enhances massage by increasing skin warmth and helping to relieve arthritic pain. Apply this topical rub to your hands and the area being massaged. Your health store or pharmacy will have a topical rub that is either scented or plain to provide a gentle, soothing action.

FOUR SELF-MASSAGE STEPS FOR ARTHRITIC
PAIN ERASURE

1. *Stroking.* Begin (and end) your massage with stroking. This is a long, sliding or stroking action of your hands along the length and grain of your muscle. Your goal is to remove the blood from the tissue and help to speed its return to the heart. NOTE: Always begin stroking at the point farthest from the heart and massage towards the heart since that is the direction you want the blood to go. REMEDY: Work-caused pain will be soothed if you use a strong, perpendicular massage or go across the grain of the muscle. This provides a circulatory as well as a conditioning effect for pain relief.

2. *Kneading.* Progress into deeper massage. Use both hands to clasp muscle, then alternate pressure from one hand to the other, squeezing and moving up the length of the muscle towards the heart. You are pressing the muscle fibers together and pushing them apart, removing the metabolic wastes. This works very well on the big muscles like thighs, calves, and upper trapezius (shoulder tops.)

3. *Friction.* Localized circular movements done around joints and tendons or around muscles. Friction is applied with fingertips, thumbs, or the fleshy base of the thumbs. The effects of friction are a spreading and broadening of the muscle fibers and a loosening and softening of ligaments and tendons around joints. Moderate pressure is applied into muscle. Move across the grain and perpendicular to the length of the muscle, or in a circular fashion. TIP: Around joints, friction should be applied without a lubricant, gently moving the skin over the underlying tissue. After friction strokes are completed, apply a topical rub to help ease joint pain.

4. *Shaking.* It is used between other techniques to relax the muscles. Use both hands on the muscles and shake back and forth in a slow, rhythmic fashion. Or loosely hold the end of a relaxed finger or toe and work it back and forth, remembering that your finger or toe extends into your hand or foot. Use large, rolling movements in shaking to loosen joint stiffness and immobility.

HOW TO SELF-MASSAGE AWAY "AFTER WORK" ARTHRITIS PAIN

Many arthritics feel pain after a day's work. A few moments of self-massage will keep muscles supple. The stimulation of soft tissues, ligaments, and tendons will help relieve "after work" arthritis pain. Here's how—

Shower first, then lie down with your legs propped up at least 45 degrees for five to ten minutes. Lie flat on the floor, and bend your left knee. Then raise your right leg and rest your right ankle on your left knee to massage your calf. Work towards your heart in massaging—always from the insertion of the muscle (the point farthest from your heart) to the origin (the point closest). NOTE: The muscle you are working on should always be relaxed. If you have to strain your back or arms in order to relax the muscle you're trying to massage, you're defeating the purpose.

Rub Away Pain

Apply the topical lotion into any painful area of the leg. For the calves, raise your knee towards your chest, resting your foot on a chair or other leg so your calf hangs loose. Begin with soft *stroking* and gradually increase the pressure of your hands. Move into the *kneading* (just like bread) phase, and become moderately more energetic with somewhat firmer hand grips. Close your eyes and try to feel the texture of the muscle. Return to *stroking* movement and slowly decrease the pressure of your work, so you ease back out of the muscle. *NEXT:* repeat in reverse.

Should Massage Be Hurtful?

You may wonder whether your self-massage should be hurtful. Any muscle with excess metabolic byproduct buildup or tension, or a joint stiffened by arthritis, may be sensitive during massage. Use common sense. Do not press too hard. Start slowly and build intensity gradually.

HOW TO RUB AWAY ARTHRITIS PAIN IN THE FEET

Begin (after a shower) by rubbing a small amount of topical lubricant onto the hurtful areas of the feet; this relieves pain and reduces friction between hands and skin.

Start on the bottom of one foot. Use your thumbs to make circular movements. *Knead* through the knots and massage the entire foot, starting with the toes and working towards the ankles. Use the pads of your fingers as tools. Squeeze the toes and then gently press the ends of the toes with the finger pads. Work your fingers between the toes and pull the toes back and forth. Then work again across the flat bottom of the foot.

Press your thumb or finger into a spot, hold for a few seconds, and then move on. Deep-stroke the arch by putting the upper hands on top of the foot and *stroking* the length of the arch with your thumbs.

Lean into your massage as best you can, so you don't wear out your fingers and arms. Use your knuckles to work around the outside edge of your heel.

Try *shaking* your toes. Remember to work up the Achilles' tendon and into your ankle. Rub around your ankle bone. Use of transverse friction massage (extending across) on the Achilles' tendon is very therapeutic to keep it pliable and strong.

Grab your foot and do a couple of ankle rotations. Then slowly flex your foot in an up-and-down movement. Work over the top and bottom of your foot with *circular friction* and finish with long *stroking* along the metatarsal bones in the foot. (They run the long way on the foot and you will feel the ridges and valleys between them.) Finish with *stroking* again and smoothing, moving towards your heart. Your feet will benefit from this pain-easing attention. So will the rest of your body!

PAIN RELIEF OF THE HANDS IN A PINCH

Self-massage of the hands is similar to that of the feet. It is extremely effective in increasing joint mobility. You can "pinch" your way to relief of hand pain in a matter of minutes.

1. Give each fingertip a good, stimulating pinch.

2. Rub each finger from tip to base and the back of your hand from each knuckle to wrist.

Remember: Always work towards, not away, from your heart.

Home Massage Remedy: Start with applying a topical lotion to any painful areas. Rub your fingertips, squeeze the ends of your fingers and wiggle. Use your thumb and forefinger. Start between fingers and press upon the sides of the knuckle joints. Move back and forth, working towards your wrist, along the ball of your hand, towards your heart. *Shake* your fingers, then *stroke.* Work along your finger bones and between them. Rub the webs between your thumb and first finger and between your other fingers.

RELIEVE ARTHRITIS PAIN IN NECK, FACE, AND HEAD

The goal of self-massage is to provide relief from tension and help alleviate everyday aches and pains. Here's how—

Apply a topical lubricant to painful areas of the neck and shoulders. *Stroke* along the tops of your shoulders, then up and down the back of your neck. Begin rubbing the muscles, going from the base of your skull down to the outside top corners of your shoulders and back up. Then work up the back of your neck to behind your ears.

Feel tight areas? They need more attention. By rubbing around and pressing into those tight spots, you can relieve arthritic tension and stiffness in your neck and shoulders.

Give Yourself a Face Rub

Before you start on your face, wash the hands thoroughly to remove all creams which should not get into or near your eyes. Apply gentle but firm pressure. With fingertips, massage your forehead, *stroking* the muscle with both hands, out from the center. Gently rub the cheeks and stroke your thumbs and fingers along the ridges of the bones surrounding the eye socket. Rub your neck and jaw line in an upward direction; apply circular friction to the ear lobes. When finishing, rub your hands together rapidly until warm, then rest your face and eyes in the palms of your hands. This is soothing and restful for your eyes.

Helpful Benefits: Self-massage helps you manage stress, promote relaxation, stimulate circulation, reduce aches and pains from muscle exertion, arthritis or tension. Remember for complete wellness, self-massage is part of your immune-rejuvenating program. It goes hand-in-hand with healthy food, sensible living habits, rest, relaxation, exercise, and a positive outlook.

When NOT to Self-Massage

Hold off self-massage after an acute injury and wait until your immune system has you on the way to recovery. Do not massage when skin is inflamed or broken. If you have any circulatory disorder, discuss massage first with your health practitioner.

RUBS AWAY PAINFUL STABS OF ARTHRITIS IN 30 MINUTES

Janet O. had agonizing, knife-like, stabbing pains in her shoulders and hands that refused to yield to conventional medications. Furthermore, she complained that drug interactions made her suffer dizzy spells, flushing, excessive sweating, and recurring bouts of gastrointestinal distress. Was she doomed to suffer ever-increasing pain that threatened to make her a cripple?

A kinesiologist (physical therapist who specializes in the mechanics and anatomy of movement with advanced training in back pain and joint distress) outlined a simple program for Janet O. that would call for 30 minutes daily of self-massage.

The goal was to "milk out" the accumulated lactic acid and other immune-defying bacteria and help restore body balance. She followed the kinesiologist's program, doubting that anything "so simple" could be effective. Happily within four days, the pains subsided and she no longer felt needle-sharp spasms. Within seven days, the self-massage had helped restore the strength of her immune system to resist hurtful invaders. She had been able to "rub away" painful arthritis . . . without drugs, and was pronounced healed by the kinesiologist. Only 30 minutes for freedom of "hopeless" arthritis!

RELIEVING PAIN AND STIFFNESS WITH
HEALING HEAT

If you have osteoarthritis, you know from experience that you can relieve soreness and stiffness by "warming up" with a little exercise. Go a bit further. You will get more benefit if you apply moist heat to sore joints as frequently as possible, whether you exercise or not.

Benefits, Limitations: Mild heat can relax tense muscles and ease muscle spasms. If you do use heat—whether in the form of a heating pad, a hot towel, or a soak in the bathtub—don't overdo it. Too much heat could worsen back spasms (not to mention cause burns). Fifteen to twenty minutes at a time is your maximum, because longer periods can tire, rather than relax, your muscles. *Caution:* Avoid using heat if you have sciatica—a painful condition caused by pressure on the sciatic nerve that runs from the lower back down the leg—because heat could aggravate this condition.

Tub Soak Warms Away Arthritis

If your entire body is affected by arthritis, simply immerse yourself in a tub of comfortably hot water (100° to 102° F.) for 15 to 20 minutes. Do this on a daily basis and your arthritis will respond with less severity as you have more mobility.

Hot Fomentation Relieves Chronic Joint Inflammation

Moist heat penetrates your skin pores and helps invigorate your immune response to "cast out" hurtful prostaglandins and bradykinin invaders. Your inflammation cools off. *Simple Remedy:* Wring out flannel strips in hot water and place them over the hurting area but *only* if you have first covered the area with a dry cloth to avoid blistering. Then cover with a strip of dry cotton. Let remain for 20 minutes. An onrush of protective cells released by your immune system will bring about a cooling of joint inflammation.

Heating Pad Helps Soothe Pain

Apply moist flannel to the aching area, then cover with a thin sheet of plastic or rubber and put a heating pad on top. Thirty minutes will be adequate for boosting immune power to help ease arthritic pain. *TIP:* You may apply comfortably hot moist towels on the area, then cover with a heating pad but *only* if it is insulated with a rubber bag. You will then enjoy the warmth for a longer amount of time.

Careful: NEVER allow yourself to go to sleep when using a heating pad. Overuse of heat dulls skin sensitivity to allow a bad burn without your being aware of it. NEVER apply heat over any skin portion that is "dead" or has impaired sensation. *Suggestion:* Have someone else in the house to be available if you doze off. Otherwise, set your alarm clock or electric timer to go off at the end of the heat treatment.

HEAT LAMP SOOTHES ARTHRITIC JOINTS

Moist heat will effectively soothe arthritic pain in the joints. Begin by applying moist towels over the affected area. Position an infrared (heat) bulb about 12 to 24 inches, depending upon

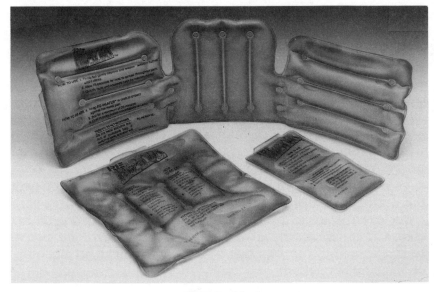

Figure 14–1

Reusable heating pack is soothing for aching areas. Your health store or pharmacy has many such products available for convenient use.

the size of the lamp. Place the lamp well above the towels and move it down until you feel a comfortable heat.

(Infrared bulbs are available in any drug store. They are *not* the same as an ultraviolet or sun lamp which you should *not* use.)

Moist heat with the help of the infrared lamp will effectively soothe pain with about 20 to 30 minutes of use. When you finish the application, cover your back with some warm flannel to protect against chilling.

HOW TO APPLY DRY HEAT

You may apply dry heat with an infrared lamp, an electric light bulb, a hot water bottle, an electric heating pad, or even a heated sand bag wrapped in dry towels. (See also Figure 14–1.) Up to 30 minutes of dry heat will effectively relieve muscle tension and help erase the spasms of pain.

OLD-FASHIONED HOT WATER BOTTLE WORKS MODERN WONDERS

The old-fashioned hot water bottle will help stimulate your blood vessels and boost immune strength to combat hurtful bacteria. Grandma may not have had modern scientific awareness but she knew it worked and that was all that mattered.

Fill a hot water bottle with hot tap water. Wrap the bottle in a strip of wool that has been soaked and wrung out in hot water. (Wear rubber gloves to protect your hands.) Cover the hurtful area with a sheet of plastic to retain heat. Apply the wrapped hot water bottle on the area and wait until it cools. Repeat several times throughout the day.

Careful: Do not use boiling hot water in the bottle since this excessive heat could penetrate the towels and cause an injury. Water that is heated to about 120° F. will do the trick.

Benefits of Moist Heat

It has a vigorous reaction on your blood circulation because it reflexly dilates the deeper-lying blood vessels; it helps relax muscles and thereby relieves pain through a healthier immune system.

SOOTHE ARTHRITIS PAIN WITH REFRESHING
COLD PACKS

Cold packs are also effective in relieving much of arthritis pain. To reduce the swelling of a joint, apply an ice pack for up to ten minutes at two-hour intervals for the first 36 hours. For chronic muscle spasms, use the ice pack for 10 to 15 minutes, two or three times a day. To protect against frostbite, keep a cloth towel between your skin and the ice pack. *Careful:* If your skin becomes white or numb, discontinue use.

Reduce Inflammation with Ice

For fast relief of inflammation and pain, apply ice for 20 minutes several times a day. Your immune system is able to stimulate a stronger blood flow. You will soon have desired results with this natural remedy.

Benefits of Ice Remedy

Cold applications help relieve aches and pains. The intense stimulation that ice provides is an excellent way to "close the gate" at the spinal pathway and inhibit painful information from reaching your brain.

Try an Ice Massage

Slowly rub the ice in circles on the spot that hurts. Do it for five to seven minutes or until the area feels numb. You can use an ice cube or a bag of frozen peas or a small package of frozen food for large areas.

Higher Altitude Helps

For leg muscles, let gravity help you. Elevate the area you're rubbing so that gravity works with you to stimulate the needed blood flow. It gives your immune system a helping boost!

Stiff Neck

Ice massage works well and fast, too. Use your fingers to find the sensitive spot on your neck and shoulder area and rub ice on it.

SPECIAL HELP FOR TRIGGER POINTS

Trigger points are irritable spots in your muscles. When a trigger point is subject to either excess emotional or physical stress, it responds by throwing a muscle into spasm which, in turn, causes pain.

Ice Remedy

An ice application erases the spasm with gentle pressure to the trigger points involved and then redirects the rebellious muscle into its normal resting relaxed condition. Here's how—

Take a single ice cube and wrap it in a hand towel. Hold it directly over your painful trigger point. Apply gently but firmly. Slowly move the cube in a circular fashion until the skin becomes ice cold. (Not a lot of pressure need be applied at this time.) When the skin gets cold, there is some natural anesthesia or dulling of pain involved.

Apply more pressure to the ice cube and below the trigger point. If it hurts, ease up on the pressure.

After ten minutes, the hot and inflamed trigger point will feel cool. Now gently massage and stretch the muscle. *Never stretch beyond the limits of comfort.*

Repeat this ice remedy once or twice a day. You will soon notice that the trigger point will release itself rather spontaneously. *Careful:* Ice should *never* be applied directly to the skin since it could cause injury.

If You Need a Cold Pack in a Hurry

Wring towels out in ice water; make a compress out of ice cubes; fill an ice bag with crushed ice. For emergency treatment of athletic injuries, coaches and trainers use chemically treated "ice bags" that work effectively. Such products are available at most health stores or pharmacies.

ICE MASSAGE COOLS INFLAMED MUSCLES

Freeze a paper cup full of water. Then remove the paper from the ice and you'll have an ice block. Put a small amount of baby oil on the skin to ease the "shock" of the cold. Then rub the ice up and down the inflamed muscular area with a firm pressure. Continue about five to ten minutes or until the skin is numbed by the cold of this ice massage.

To protect your hands from the cold, you could wear rubber gloves. Otherwise, insert an ice cream stick into the cup so that when the water is frozen, you hold onto the stick instead of the ice. Certain types of muscular inflammation will be relieved with this easy, do-it-yourself ice massage. (Should pain return when the cold effects wear off, repeat again.)

HOW CONTRAST BATHS WAKE UP YOUR SLUGGISH IMMUNE SYSTEM

Alternating heat and cold applications (also known as contrast baths although no tub soaking is necessary) will help stimulate your immune system to "flush out" hurtful impurities that have penetrated your protective barrier. An increase in blood circulation will further provide a stronger resistance to recurring discomfort.

You Will Need: Two plastic (or rubber) containers. (One is filled with hot tap water; the other is filled with ice cubes or crushed ice.) Hand towels. Hot water bottle. Follow this program:

1. Place a comfortably hot, moist towel over the aching area. Then put a hot water bottle filled with the hot tap water on top of the moist towel. Let remain for 15 minutes.

2. Place a comfortably cold, moist towel over the same aching area. Then put another towel, which has wrapped ice cubes within, on top of the moist towel. Let remain for five minutes.

3. Alternate the hot-cold applications five times.

Remember: Begin with the hot application, finish with the hot application. You may need to refill the hot water bottle between applications so that it remains hot; the ice cubes may be put in another bottle for longer lasting results. Otherwise, wrap in a towel.

Suggestion: You may simplify the contrast bath by wringing towels out in hot water and cold water. If so, your hot water should not be above 125° F. Your cold water should be 55° F. or lower.

The "contrast" of hot and cold will give a beneficial boost to your immune system to "chase out" irritants and viral enemies.

CHASES ARTHRITIS AWAY WITH HOME WATER TREATMENTS

Late one afternoon when Henry T. unloaded his last sack of potatoes from the back of his station wagon, he experienced a sharp, stabbing pain in the lumbar (lower) region of his back. As a truck farmer, he was more than 50 miles from the nearest hospital. He managed to drive home, hunched over the wheel, but the pain persisted to the extent that shooting needle-points were stabbing down the backs of his legs.

He spent a sleepless night, hardly able to turn over in bed. At daybreak, the throbbing pain was so severe, he walked with a limp. He always had varying degrees of arthritis, but this outbreak threatened to immobilize him. His wife was friends with a neighboring farm woman whose son was a physical therapist. He was speedily summoned. He outlined a program for Henry T. which included hot applications and cold applications but emphasized the need for the contrasting baths. They were to begin at once.

The truck farmer was desperate since he wanted to avoid surgery. He began the hydrotherapy remedies immediately. Within three days, he could walk with a healthy posture as the shooting needles "went away." After nine days of the water treatments, he had so recovered, he could return to his truck farming with the flexibility of years ago. *Special Bonus:* Henry T. no longer felt "former arthritis" pain that was also "cast out" with the help of the hydrotherapy!

Arthritis Relief at Your Fingertips

You can revitalize your immune system to protect your body against painful arthritis with your fingertips. Whether a soothing massage or various do-it-yourself water applications, help is available. If you have been caught up in a revolving door routine in seeking help, look to immunotherapy as a potential solution to the problem of arthritis. It is as close as your fingertips!

IN REVIEW

1. Pain is a reaction to a weakness in your immune system, crying for speedy help.
2. Self-massage helps block painful bradykinin substances and "switches off" pain in a matter of minutes.
3. Feel a pain or generalized stiffness? Find relief with the four self-massage steps. They erase pain swiftly.
4. Rub away foot and leg pain with easy massage motions in the privacy of your home.
5. Relieve pain and stiffness with healing heat. Tub soaks, cloth applications, and hydrotherapy stimulate the healing power of your immune system to overcome arthritis infections.
6. Give yourself an ice rub and feel pains vanish in minutes.
7. Janet O. rubbed away painful arthritis stabs in 30 minutes with self-massage.
8. Henry T. chased away "near crippling" arthritis with home water treatments.

15

Correct Your Posture and Cast Out Arthritis

The spine is not an inflexible rod as some people would believe. In fact, it is quite flexible. Although structurally strong, it reflects the vigorous movement of the human body. It not only supports the body and all its organs, it also moves constantly. Every activity, even breathing, demands movement of the spine and ribs and attachments. The spine gives the human structure both strength and agility. Yet it can be abused with improper posture which could reduce immune protection and predispose to arthritis.

Be Alert to Spinal Abuse

Modern people, as a group, have neglected what Nature has so skillfully provided. Through misuse and non-use—through too much sitting, not enough exercise, too much daily stress and other bad habits—you allow your back, buttocks, and abdominal muscles to become both too weak and too tense. A back whose supporting muscles have lost their strength and flexibility is a vulnerable back. It is liable to endure immune breakdowns that are felt through the mechanism of pain.

Spine, Arthritis, Pain

As you reach the middle years, your bones tend to change slightly in response to a lifetime of wear and tear. Our vertebrae (bones in the back) may flatten out somewhat and develop

189

rough edges and protruding spurs of bone. Sometimes these spurs irritate the spinal cord or the nerves that branch from the spine. A spur often causes such intense pain that surgery may be considered. But arthritis of the spine is usually too diffuse and the pain not serious enough to warrant surgery. A fitness program to help boost the vigor of the immune system will slow down the erosion process, reduce the symptoms, and extend the prime of life of the spinal column.

PRACTICAL STEPS TO HEALTHY POSTURE

Correct posture will build immunity to pain and stiffness, improve breathing, and keep joints flexible. Basic steps are:

Stand with your shoulders, hips, and knees straight, stomach in, and head held high.

Walk with your arms swinging freely and your weight shifting from side to side as you walk. TIP: To prevent your muscles from tiring too quickly, avoid carrying heavy packages.

Sit whenever you can. Standing needlessly will cause you to tire easily. Sit in a firm chair that is not too low, has a straight back and armrests. TIP: When you are sitting, keep your shoulders back, head up, stomach in, and feet flat on the floor.

Sleep on a firm mattress. A plywood board at least 1/2 inch thick and the same size as the mattress placed between the bedspring and mattress will keep it from sagging. When lying down or sleeping, try to lie flat on your back. If you use a pillow, it should be a small one. Knees and hips should be straight. Arms and hands should be straightened out at your side—not folded over your body. Never place a pillow under your knees.

Healthy posture calls for simple efforts to stand straight in a comfortable and semi-relaxed position; there should be no strain on muscles, joints, or ligaments. In this way, you will be good to your spinal column and help resist the onset of arthritic disorders.

A STRAIGHT SPINE BUILDS IMMUNITY TO ARTHRITIS

It is important to sit, stand, and sleep in positions that do not allow your joints to stiffen in a bent or deformed position. If you have arthritis symptoms in your spinal region, make every effort to keep your spine straight and erect at all times. If you are a desk or bench worker, avoid slumping or you may weaken your immune system and eventually be unable to thoroughly straighten up.

TOO MUCH SITTING CAN BE A PAIN IN THE BACK

Improper sitting posture could lead to arthritic pain. But even if you sit properly, too much of it could be hurtful to your hips, knees, and elbows.

Immune Problem: Prolonged joint flexion weakens the immune system by allowing muscle shortening and joint adhesions to block extension of the joints. If your hip muscles shorten in a sitting position, they react with a tug on your spinal column so that you start to slump. Gradually, the pull of gravity bends your spine into a bow. Your distorted immune system becomes weak and arthritis infection can seize hold.

Immune Solution: If your situation calls for much sitting, be sure to maintain correct sitting posture at all times. Take frequent "standing" breaks throughout the day. Stand on your toes, extend both arms high over your head, reach for the sky, try to pluck stars out of the heavens! Only ten minutes of this "standing" break every hour or so will help stimulate your immune system to strengthen your spinal column to resist arthritis.

DO YOU SIT WITH A "C" SHAPE OR AN "S" SHAPE?

Chairs, sofas, and office furniture were not designed for human beings. There is a tendency to flop into a seat, throwing the back into a drooping "C" shape. Instead, you would have a stronger immune-stimulating spinal column if you sat in an "S" shape. Note the differences and benefits:

"C" Shape. This puts excessive stretch on the lower or lumbar ligaments, while compressing or impinging on the outlet of nerves through the spinal column. It irritates the flexor withdrawal holding pattern.

"S" Shape. This is the healthful posture you assume during standing or walking. Find a chair that allows you to use a small pillow, perhaps 2 to 3 inches thick, based at the small of your back. By projecting your abdomen slightly forward, with the lower part of the "S"-shaped curve being supported, your neck and shoulders will fall into line; your head will not be thrust forward but will be held back properly on your shoulders without strain.

Check Your Reading Posture

So much of neck and shoulder arthritis pain is related to hanging over a book or work at a desk in such a way that the muscles in the back of the neck and shoulders have to hold the head up continuously. The muscles tend to contract tighter throughout the day, filling the trigger points and throwing you into arthritic spasm by evening.

Healthy Reading Posture: While you are reading this book, improve your holding pattern. Let your head rest on your shoulders in such a way that if it were to fall, it could fall backwards as easily as it could tilt forward or to either side. In other words, it should be *balanced* on your shoulders, so that no muscle group is required to stay painfully contracted for long periods of time.

Check Your Driving Posture

The above problems with seating apply doubly to driving an automobile, especially if you have had mishaps. You tend to drive with a lot more vigilance and tension when you know the potential damage a car wreck can cause.

Healthy Driving Posture: Insert a small pillow at the small of your back, as well as a wedged pillow of about 2-inch thickness at your buttocks. You will be able to rotate your pelvis forward as you drive your car—thus maintaining the "S"-shaped curve in your back. This helps keep your shoulders back farther towards the seat of of your car, allowing your head to rest comfortably thereon.

Relaxation Protects Against Pain

Many people drive when they're particularly sleepy or tired (going to or from work). During these times, you have a tendency to thrust your head forward, producing greater strain on your neck and shoulder muscles. A remedy is to listen to soothing and quiet music as you commute; it allows a transition point— a private moment to help you face the activities ahead. Try using a soothing, melodic cassette tape, instead of listening to the hectic morning news and see how different your neck and shoulder muscles feel by the time you reach your destination.

EYESIGHT, DISTANCE, POSTURE

Even such a seemingly minor thing as the focal length of your glasses is an exceedingly important part of your postural support system. If you normally read a page some 8 to 10 inches from your eyes, you need to thrust your head and jaw forward. This distorts your spinal column and weakens your immune response to pain and arthritis.

Remedy: Have your vision specialist remake your glasses so that the focal length averages between 12 and 16 inches. You will then be able to read without putting excessive pressure on your neck muscles. If you wear bifocals, your visual field is frequently even more constricted. Having glasses made so that eye movements can remain comfortably unimpeded is helpful in keeping your neck muscle tone in good shape.

So often, it is not a refractive error or disease within the eye that causes arthritic pains of the head and neck; it is simply inappropriate focal length adjustment in glasses. Remember that folks who wear glasses have to track what they read with very minute and highly tuned movements of the neck because their field of vision is narrower than those who do not wear glasses.

Since trigger points occur in areas within muscles of maximum functional binding and least movement, it is important to determine if your ways of movement are symmetrical enough to avoid binding up your muscles.

HOW TO SLEEP CORRECTLY TO BOOST IMMUNE RESPONSE TO ARTHRITIS

So-called morning stiffness, afternoon bursitis, or evening low back pain could be traced to unhealthy sleeping posture the night before. You have abused your immune system and your aching muscles and spinal column react with poor posture as well as bedding. Simple corrective steps include:

A Firm Mattress

In bed, your back muscles relax. Your spinal ligaments assume the obligation of holding the vertebrae in proper alignment. If your bed sags, much strain is placed on your spinal joints and ligaments which weakens your immune system. You may insert a ½-inch thick sheet of plywood between mattress and springs to firm up your bed. Available are innerspring mattresses that mold themselves to your body contours and support your spine in a level, horizontal position.

THE BEST SLEEPING POSITION

To maintain proper spinal alignment—*sleep on your back.* Use a thin pillow (or no pillow) beneath your head so your neck remains in line with your spine. Feel pain in your lower back when reclining? Place a thin pillow beneath both knees. This eases any strain. Try *not* to sleep with hands folded over your stomach. This causes a temporary numbness on the small finger side of your hand and forearm because of pressure against the ulnar nerve in your elbow. TIP: Change the position of your arms. Insert a soft pillow under each elbow to ease such hurts upon the immune system.

STOMACH SLEEPER? THAT'S A "NO-NO"

Sleeping face down causes a back as well as shoulder and stomach curvature that could give you morning stiffness and an arthritic outrage. If you cannot control stomach sleeping, do not use any pillow under your head. To ease lower back distress, bend one knee up and out on the side toward which your face is turned. TIP: A thin pillow inserted beneath the edge of your front side stomach will protect against much spinal sag.

Sleeping on Your Side

Insert a thick pillow beneath your head and bend both knees. To protect against back trouble, put the pillow between your knees so that both thighs will rest parallel to each other. If you have a narrow waist but heavy hips, insert a thin pillow beneath your side so that your spine will not sag when you lie on your side.

For arthritics with low back distress, you will rest most comfortably if you lie flat on your back with good spinal support.

CORRECTS BAD POSTURE AND CORRECTS ARTHRITIS WITHOUT PILLS

Retired bus driver, Arthur V., complained he was so stiff with arthritis in the morning, he could scarcely move. He was given stronger and stronger doses of "pain pills" that gave him headaches and bouts with colitis while easing his discomfort to a mild degree.

When examined by a physiatrist (an M. D. with extensive training in the treatment of disabilities and more directed toward immune rebuilding through physical rehabilitation and hydrotherapy), Arthur V. was told that with a change in sleeping as well as daily posture, he might boost his immune system resistance to arthritis recurrence.

Proper mattress and improved sleeping, reading, and walking postures worked so effectively, he was relieved from his painful arthritis in 11 days. He threw out his "pain pills" along with his too-soft mattress and was so energetic, he decided to work part-time!

LOSE EXCESS WEIGHT AND LOSE ARTHRITIS

There is no question that excess body weight aggravates arthritis. With a weakening of the immune system, infection occurs via a biomechanical, chemical, or metabolic reaction.

Surplus pounds cause more strain on bones, joints, and muscles—particularly the cartilage joint surfaces affected by arthritis.

Normal cartilage is compressible. The joint space decreases to about one-half its resting height when you stand. Excess body weight causes serious compression of the cartilage and does not give sufficient recovery time for normal circulation which lowers your immune response. This wears away joint surfaces. Such wear and tear reduces the life and health of the joint.

Stress, Strain, Sickness

Excess weight puts stress and strain on your ligaments and tendons during walking, bending, climbing steps, lifting, and carrying. It shreds your immune system and paves the way to sickness via muscle fatigue. An extra demand is made on the circulation for needed immune nutrients such as oxygen and glycogen. The length of time needed by the muscles, bones, and joints for rest and recuperation is considerably increased. Excess fat is also a threat to the health of your arteries and circulatory system. For the arthritic, obesity is a constant and painful threat.

Slim Down, Improve Immunity, Heal Arthritis

Shed excess weight and your immune system is subjected to less abuse (along with your body). Better nourishment helps resist the onrush of arthritis invaders and healing is all the more possible.

OSTEOPOROSIS—"THIN BONES"

The bones of the body, like other tissues and organs, are constantly being repaired with minerals and other nutrients to keep them strong. By middle age, the body may do this less efficiently; at some point, for some people, the bones do not retain the nutrients they need to stay solid and strong. They become less dense, more brittle and thin, a condition called osteoporosis. Vertebrae weakened by osteoporosis may collapse under the normal weight of the body.

Over a million bone fractures each year, widespread disability, and billions of dollars in health care expenses might be prevented by boosting the immune system of middle-aged women to protect against osteoporosis. (See Figure 15–1.)

Who Is at Risk?

Some women are at greater risk than others after reaching middle age. These include women who are thin or petite (i.e., small-boned), smoke, abuse alcohol, have a diet low in calcium, exercise very little, or use certain medications such as corticosteroids.

Is Nutrition Important?

Your immune system protects against thin bones if your body has enough calcium to sustain mass and strength. Dairy products are a good source of dietary calcium. Sardines, broccoli, and leafy green vegetables are also good sources of calcium. (High-fat cheeses and whole milk contain too much saturated fat which is linked to cardiovascular disease, so either limit or else switch to low-fat or non-fat dairy products.) A glass of milk or a cup of non-fat yogurt has 300 milligrams of calcium. Immunologists suggest 1,500 milligrams daily. You may prefer calcium supplements. Which ones?

Simple Test: Place the supplement in 6 ounces of white vinegar at room temperature for 30 minutes, stirring occasionally. If it dissolves speedily, it will do the same in your system for rapid use by your immune system.

Vitamin D Is Needed

Most milk products have added Vitamin D which works with calcium to build strong bones. Otherwise, only 20 minutes a day in the sunshine will supply sufficient amounts of this vitamin.

Exercise Boosts Immune Response to Osteoporosis

Weight-bearing exercises such as walking or jogging for 30 to 60 minutes, five times a week, will boost immune response to help increase bone size and strength. Your bones need the tug and pull of regular muscular action so your immune system can keep them healthy and control or prevent excessive calcium loss. *Note:* Any exercise program should be undertaken by

Bone Damage After Menopause

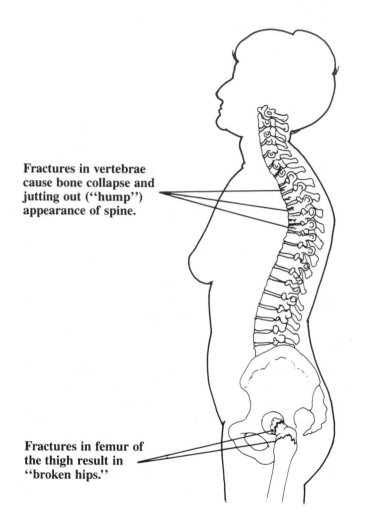

Fractures in vertebrae cause bone collapse and jutting out ("hump") appearance of spine.

Fractures in femur of the thigh result in "broken hips."

COURTESY — THE UPJOHN COMPANY

Bone depletion due to loss of female hormones after menopause results in an estimated 1.3 million fractures a year. Spinal fractures contribute to a loss of height and hunched-over posture. Hip fractures can cause disability as well as death.

Figure 15–1

women whose health practitioners consider them suitable candidates.

TEN EASY EXERCISES TO IMPROVE POSTURE AND EASE ARTHRITIS

Your immune system functions with the help of oxygen and nutrition via a healthy circulatory system. Give your immune system the "breath of life" by invigorating your body with simple exercises. The following set of ten exercises will wake up your sluggish circulation, ease arthritis distress, and improve your basic posture. Your immune system threshold is raised and you will have a stronger resistance to outside invaders. *Suggestion:* Never strain or allow yourself to feel hurt. Obtain approval from your health practitioner for these and any other exercises.

#1. Raise your arms over your head as high as you can, elbows straight. Then swing arms out, down, and around in a big circle. Repeat five times.

#2. Place hands behind your head. Gently move elbows back as far as they will go and simultaneously pull your chin in and head back. Repeat five times.

#3. Grasp the handle of a medium-weight hammer close to its head. Keep upper arm by your side with elbow bent to a right angle. Turn wrist from left to right, letting weight of hammer swing hand over as far as possible each time. (As you improve, move your grip farther down the handle so that the hammer's weight makes you work a bit harder.) Repeat five times.

#4. Place hand flat on table. Spread fingers apart keeping them straight. Lift index finger. Then lift all fingers and thumb— while palm remains pressed down. Finally, lift fingers, thumb, and hand, bending wrist up as far as possible—while you keep your forearm on the table. Repeat five times.

#5. Open your hand, spreading your fingers as you do. Close, making as tight a fist as possible. After repeating this several times, touch tip of each thumb to each finger, pinching firmly each time and forming a letter "O". Repeat five times.

#6. Lie comfortably on your back. Bend knee and hip up toward chest as far as possible. Lower leg slowly, straightening knee as you go. Repeat five times.

#7. Lie comfortably flat on your back, legs straight and about 6 inches apart. Point toes toward each other. Move right leg out to side, return. Move left leg out to side, return. Keep toes pointed toward each other. Repeat five times.

#8. Sit in a chair. Keep feet flat on the floor. Raise toes as high as you can but keep heels on the floor. Then reverse, keeping toes down but lifting heels as high as you can. Finally, with both feet flat, lift inside of each foot and roll its weight over on the outside—keeping the toes curled down. Repeat five times.

#9. Take ten very deep breaths. Exhale. Now lie flat on your stomach, arms down by your sides. Lift head and bend your knees at the same time—as far as comfortably possible. If you can, lift your knees a little. Repeat five times.

#10. Lie on your back, knees straight. Lift your head, curling your back forward into a sitting position, hands reaching out to your toes. Lie back down. Repeat five times.

"HOPELESS" ARTHRITIS BECOMES "HEALED" WITH IMMUNE ALERT

Overweight waitress and part-time restaurant cook, Helen McC., felt her joints were "freezing" and her arms were "heavy" until it was difficult to write down a customer's order, let alone work in the kitchen. Her arthritis was threatening her existence. Medications caused such a diuretic effect, she became nutritionally deficient. She was developing osteoporosis to compound the arthritis syndrome. Yet if she skipped a pill, the hurt and some inflammation returned so that her movements were painfully restricted. She was caught up in a vicious circle.

A highly recommended osteopath (licensed physician with special training in manipulation therapy and nutrition) took tests and immediately diagnosed a weakening of the immune system traced to: overweight, poor oxygen supply, weak circulation, and calcium deficiency. He suggested a low-fat, low-calorie diet along with a set of the preceding ten exercises that took less than 30 minutes each day. He also suggested 1,500 milligrams of calcium from food and/or supplements.

Helen McC. was astonished because her formerly "hopeless" arthritis began to respond as pounds melted and flexibility was restored. She made one psychological change: no more work in an eating place where food could be too tempting. She was "healed" of her arthritis within seven weeks. Gone were her pains along with her medications. Her immune system was alerted to keep her alive!

A Strong Skeleton Is a Powerful Immune Barrier to Arthritis

Maintain a strong and healthy posture. The way you stand, walk, sit, and sleep *does* influence your resistance to arthritis and its elimination, too. A healthy posture will give you a healthy, arthritis-resisting immune system. Be good to your spine! Your immune system will be grateful!

IN REVIEW

1. Spinal abuse could weaken your immune system and pre-dispose your body to arthritis. Correct your posture for stronger resistance to infectious invaders.
2. Note the basic postural improvement steps to better health. Easy, effective, healing.
3. Change your sitting posture from a "C" shape to an "S" shape and ease the strain of arthritis in minutes.
4. Check your reading and driving and sleeping postures. Simple changes may well reverse and eradicate arthritis distress.
5. Arthur V. stimulated his immune system with correct sleeping positions and was able to wake up—free of arthritis!
6. Lose excess weight and ease joint strain for reduction in symptoms. Your immune system functions youthfully if you are slim.
7. Nutrition plus exercise helps guard against the bone-thinning threat of osteoporosis.
8. A set of ten easy exercises revitalize your body's skeleton and restore function and vigor to your arthritis-fighting immune system.
9. Helen McC. went from "hopeless" to "healed" when an immune alert program speedily eliminated her arthritis syndrome.

16

How Exercise Strengthens the Immune System to Heal Arthritis

The invasion of arthritis is affected by a number of factors, primary of which is your physical condition. Its progress almost exactly parallels the condition of your immune system and the competence of the cells that make up that system. To protect against the onset and increase of arthritis, you need to bolster your immune response.

Exercise and Immune Power

Daily exercises may well be the strongest medicine you need to ease the symptoms of arthritis. Exercise not only strengthens your bones, muscles, heart, and lungs, but also increases the potency of your immune system. It makes every body cell function better—in particular, the white blood cells which are needed in the fight against arthritis.

Endorphins, Pain Control, Arthritis Healing

During activity, your body releases endorphins, those magical substances emitted from the brain. These endorphins circulate throughout your body to soothe pain and bring about a healing of arthritis. During physical activity, a higher demand for oxygen causes blood vessels to expand throughout the body in order to deliver more oxygenated blood. *Benefit:* This increase in blood flow is beneficial because the cells of the immune system must also travel in the bloodstream. As the delivery of these arthritis-soothing agents improves, so does their healing reaction.

Whole Body Healing with Exercise

Regular exercise revitalizes the metabolic processes including digestion, absorption, and elimination. The transfer of healing nutrients into body tissues is speedily enhanced, as is the elimination of arthritis-causing poisons through your liver, skin, and kidneys. Exercise also lowers the resting cardiac and respiratory rates; this helps conserve the energy you need to overcome your arthritis.

Exercise also improves your mental attitude, providing you with powerful psychological strength that is so valuable in maintaining a strong immune system. Exercise is one of the most positive and beneficial therapies that can be blended into an adjunct program.

Helps Strengthen Bone Structure

Troubled with "thin bones" even if you take calcium? This mineral is better absorbed if you keep active. Walking, jogging, hiking, aerobics, tennis and golf are great weight-bearing exercises that boost calcium absorption into the bones.

Exercise further strengthens muscles and increases bone mass, improving balance and agility, thereby helping to prevent falls. It's *never* too late to benefit from exercise! Women past 80 in nursing homes have revitalized the immune system and been able to increase the density of their bones over other women who are more sedentary.

Walk Away Arthritis Pain

When you walk, the outpouring of endorphin will soothe pain. Your immune system is able to help shield you from excessive pain with a brisk walk of only 30 to 40 minutes. It's Nature's most favorite "pain killer."

EXERCISE, BONE STRENGTH, BODY REVITALIZATION

Generally, exercise is good for everyone! It helps you look and feel better. It provides you with more energy, helps you sleep better, and also helps control weight. Walking and swimming are good for the heart because they improve endurance and blood flow and can decrease hardening of the arteries to enable T-cells free movement to boost immunity.

Exercise melts stress and depression. It leads to an improved sense of self-esteem and accomplishment. In addition, exercising with a friend or being part of a class is a good way to socialize.

Why Exercise Is Needed by Bones

To understand why, it is helpful to know about the structure of the joints. In brief, a *joint* is the place in the body where two bones come together. *Bone* is living tissue that can grow and rebuild (for example, when a broken bone heals.) *Movement helps keep your bones strong.* When you are inactive, your bones lose calcium and become brittle.

The ends of the bones are covered with *cartilage.* This is tough, elastic tissue that cushions and protects the bone ends. Easy, smooth movement is necessary to nourish your cartilage.

Insufficient Movement = Weakened Immune System

When you do not move enough, your joints become stiff, your muscles become weaker and smaller as your immune system becomes inadequate. *Problem:* If you have a painful joint, you often keep the joint in a bent position because it feels better that way. If the joint stays bent too long it can become locked. Loss of function of that joint and deformity can result. *Solution:* Invigorate your immune system with regular exercises to help move your joints more easily. The outpouring of pain-easing endorphins and infection-fighting white blood cells further help promote healing.

GETTING STARTED IN EXERCISE

How to determine what kind of exercise to do? First of all, discuss it with your health practitioner if you have varying degrees of arthritis. You may need to do specifically prescribed exercises.

Stay within your own limits. Avoid hurt! Don't try to "test" yourself by choosing any activity that is too hard or too stressful for your body. If you would feel better in a group exercise program, ask your practitioner for suggestions. *Note:* A fitness program should be recreation and *also* therapeutic!

WHEN TO EXERCISE

1. Find a specific time and place. Basically, it is best to exercise when you have the least pain and stiffness; when you are not tired. *Tip:* You might try exercising at different times of the day until you decide what is best for you. Some folks have found that exercise reduces their morning stiffness.

2. Exercise daily. If you miss a few sessions, you will need to start again at a slightly lower level. If you must miss a day, just get back into the routine and focus on the progress you'll be making toward your goal.

3. Don't exercise on a full stomach if you find it uncomfortable. Wait at least two hours after a meal.

HOW TO PREPARE

If pain and stiffness are a problem for you, prepare for exercises by massaging the affected area, or by applying heat or cold, or both heat and cold.

Heat

It relaxes joints and muscles and helps to relieve pain. Taking a warm (not hot) shower just before the exercise session may help you do the exercises more easily. Also, there are other methods of heat (electric blanket, whirlpools, hot packs) that you can try. Use the one that is most effective and convenient for you. Whatever method you choose, make sure you are using it correctly. Only mild heat is necessary to get results. It should feel soothing and comfortable, not hot. You will get the full benefit of heat by using it for about 20 minutes each time.

Cold

Some folks prefer cold to reduce pain in specific joints. You can make a cold pack by filling a plastic bag with crushed ice. Or, try wrapping a package of frozen vegetables in a towel. Place the cold pack over the painful joint with a towel in between. You will receive the most benefit in 10 to 15 minutes.

Both Heat and Cold

Some people find relief by using a combination of heat and cold. To do this, you alternate warm- and cold-water applications. This is called a contrast bath. Soak your hands or feet in warm water (about 110° F.) for about three minutes. Then soak them in a container of cold water (about 65° F.) for one minute. Repeat this process three times. End the treatment with a warm-water soak.

Warm Up—Cool Down

When doing any kind of vigorous exercise, be sure to first "warm up." *Begin activity at a very slow pace and increase gradually.* At the end of your exercise session, "cool down" by slowing your rate of movement and allowing your breathing and heart rate to return to normal. Do gentle stretching exercises as part of warming up and cooling down. This will help you to avoid injury and to reduce the chance of being stiff or sore the next day. It will also increase your enjoyment of the activity!

What to Wear

Loose, comfortable clothing. Shoes should provide good support. Make sure the soles of your shoes are made of non-slip material.

HOW TO CARRY OUT EXERCISES

1. If you've been inactive for a long time, it will take a while to get into shape. Begin doing each exercise a few times. Gradually increase the number of repetitions.

2. Exercise with a slow, steady rhythm, giving your muscles time to relax between each repetition. Don't try to hurry. It is

more important to perform the motion slowly and completely rather than increasing speed and number of repetitions.

3. Coordinate your breathing with the exercises. Do *not* hold your breath. Counting your exercises out loud will help you breathe deeply and regularly.

4. If a joint is hot and inflamed (red, swollen, painful), move it *gently* through its available range of motion. Seek help from your practitioner if you need to adapt your exercises or must make changes when you are having a flare-up.

PRACTICAL GUIDELINES FOR COMFORT AND HEALING

1. Remember that arthritis symptoms come and go. Exercises that seem easy one day may be too hard the next. When this happens, cut back on the number of exercises and then add more when you can.

2. Wear warm clothing and avoid becoming chilled while exercising. Cold drafts in the dressing and/or exercise room can lead to muscle tension. If you are exercising in a pool, the water temperature should be 83 to 88 degrees.

3. Stop exercising immediately if you: have any chest tightness or chest pain, severe shortness of breath, or feel dizzy, faint, or sick to your stomach. If symptoms continue contact your practitioner.

4. If you have a muscle pain or cramping during any exercise, stop that exercise. Relax the affected muscle and gently rub it with your hands. Continue with slow exercise and easier movements.

5. Read your body's signals that tell you of your immune response: increased depth and rate of breathing; increased heart rate; mild to moderate sweating; feeling or hearing your heart beat; mild muscle aches and tenderness during the first weeks of exercise.

6. Exercise should cause only minimal stress on your joints. Avoid weight-lifting unless personally prescribed. It is best to move your joints by yourself. If you need help, ask your practitioner.

7. Be careful not to overdo it. If you still have pain (as a result of exercising) two hours after you've stopped, or if your symptoms are worse the next day in the joints you have exercised, then you've done too much. As a general rule: If you start having sharp pain or more pain than is usual with your exercise—*stop!* Pain is a warning signal. Using hot, swollen joints *too much* will weaken your immune system and cause further injury. The next time, decrease the number of times you do each exercise, or do them more gently. If these steps don't help, find a different exercise that will achieve the same result that is more suitable for you.

8. Remember that group exercise programs are usually *not* designed to be therapeutic. They do not take the place of exercises that may have been prescribed for you by your health practitioner.

Yes, exercise is important to boost immune healing power to help you decrease pain and stiffness. To begin, here is a set of nine simple exercises that will start the flow of pain-relieving endorphins and also boost your immune response to induce healing benefits.

Instructions for Exercises

(1) Do these once or twice daily to maintain joint mobility. (2) Move in a slow, steady manner. Do not bounce. (3) A gentle stretch at the end of each motion is okay, but there should be no pain. (4) Make sure you breathe regularly as you exercise. *Do not hold your breath.* You may want to count out loud. (5) Do each repetition five to ten times. (See Figure 16–1 for exercises.)

REVERSES TIDE OF HURTFUL ARTHRITIS
VIA EXERCISE

His shoulder arthritis was spreading until it was difficult for him to get in and out of tight areas such as his automobile. Jason R. M. was concerned over the slow but steady increase in joint stiffness and recurring flareups of inflammation in his wrists and fingers. Was he going to become handicapped?

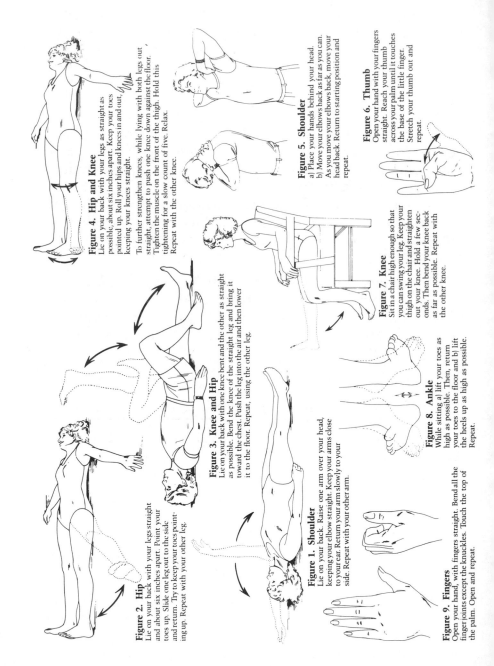

Figure 4. Hip and Knee

Lie on your back with your legs as straight as possible, about six inches apart. Keep your toes pointed up. Roll your hips and knees in and out, keeping your knees straight.

To further strengthen knees, while lying with both legs out straight, attempt to push one knee down against the floor. Tighten the muscle on the front of the thigh. Hold this tightening for a slow count of five. Relax. Repeat with the other knee.

Figure 5. Shoulder

a) Place your hands behind your head.
b) Move your elbows back as far as you can. As you move your elbows back, move your head back. Return to starting position and repeat.

Figure 6. Thumb

Open your hand with your fingers straight. Reach your thumb across your palm until it touches the base of the little finger. Stretch your thumb out and repeat.

Figure 7. Knee

Sit in a chair high enough so that you can swing your leg. Keep your thigh on the chair and straighten out your knee. Hold a few seconds. Then bend your knee back as far as possible. Repeat with the other knee.

Figure 2. Hip

Lie on your back with your legs straight and about six inches apart. Point your toes up. Slide one leg out to the side and return. Try to keep your toes pointing up. Repeat with your other leg.

Figure 3. Knee and Hip

Lie on your back with one knee bent and the other as straight as possible. Bend the knee of the straight leg and bring it toward the chest. Push the leg into the air and then lower it to the floor. Repeat, using the other leg.

Figure 8. Ankle

While sitting a) lift your toes as high as possible. Then, return your toes to the floor and b) lift the heels up as high as possible. Repeat.

Figure 1. Shoulder

Lie on your back. Raise one arm over your head, keeping your elbow straight. Keep your arms close to your ear. Return your arm slowly to your side. Repeat with your other arm.

Figure 9. Fingers

Open your hand, with fingers straight. Bend all the finger joints except the knuckles. Touch the top of the palm. Open and repeat.

Figure 16–1

A complete patient history conducted by an orthopedist (specialist in disorders of the musculoskeletal system which includes bones, muscles, joints, ligaments, and tendons) brought to light a sluggish immune system. Jason R. M. was a sedentary person, rarely walking more than absolutely necessary. He even had a remote control television set so he could sit for hours and switch channels without getting up.

The orthopedist suggested he walk more and sit less. He also prescribed the preceding nine range-of-motion exercises to breathe "new life into a tired immune system." Jason R. M. was told to give up the remote control TV. More movement meant a stronger immune system. He followed the exercise program and became more physically active. Within three weeks, his stiffness was gone. His inflammation cooled off and he was soon free of the symptoms. He celebrated by joining a jogging club . . . and became a winner!

IMMUNE-INVIGORATING EXERCISES YOU CAN DO ANYWHERE

First, each exercise should be done with a *mild* stretch sensation. No pain. No breath-holding.

ELBOW SWINGS—Sit on a chair, keeping back straight and feet flat on the floor. Bend arms at elbow and hold them at your side. Push shoulders back as far as comfortably possible, then return to starting position and repeat.

POSTURE CORRECTION—Stand straight with back against wall. Place elbows against wall. Press them gently backward while pinching shoulder blades together. Slowly release and repeat while keeping erect posture.

SHOULDER SHRUGS—Keep arms straight and at sides while you raise shoulders up, forward, and down. Repeat exercise by raising shoulders up, backward, and down.

LATERAL SHIFT—Stand with feet shoulder-width apart and arms straight out (like a scarecrow). Shift hips from side to side. Do not bend over sideways.

WALL ARCH—Stand facing the wall with arms stretched up and toes touching the wall. Then, move feet backward while keeping arms and chest in contact with the wall, ending with back in its deeper *comfortable* arch.

TRUNK TWISTS—Position legs shoulder-width apart and arms straight out (scarecrow position). Gently turn upper torso to either side.

DEEP BREATHING—Stand straight with arms at sides. Inhale while raising arms and stretching them over your head. Exhale while slowly bringing arms down to your side and repeat.

BONE-STRENGTHENING EXERCISES

ARM CIRCLES—With arms held straight out (scarecrow position), alternate small and large circles in both directions.

WALL-SLIDE—Lean back against wall, placing feet shoulder-width apart. Gently bend knees down a few inches, keeping back against the wall. Raise up and repeat.

SIDE LEG LIFTS—Lie on side while supporting head in bottom hand. Raise top leg up and down while keeping knee straight. Turn on other side and repeat.

HEAD RAISES—Lie on back with knees bent and hands on stomach. Slowly raise your head a few inches while keeping shoulders in contact with the floor. Gently lower your head and repeat.

KICK-UPS—Kneel on hands and knees, locking elbows. Lift one leg up and back, bending at the knee. Do not raise your knee above hip-line. Lower leg to the starting position and repeat, alternating legs.

HAND-SQUEEZE—With arms held straight out (scarecrow position), look forward while clenching and unclenching fists.

PRESS-UPS—Start by lying down in "push-up" position. While straightening arms, arch lower back, pinching shoulder blades together. Slowly return to starting position and repeat.

SIDE KNEE BENDS—Lie on side while supporting head in bottom hand. Draw top leg toward head while bending knee, then return to start position and repeat. Turn on either side and repeat.

PELVIC TILTS—Lie on your back with knees bent. Gently press lower back down flat on floor. Release and then gently arch lower back while keeping buttocks on floor.

INDOOR FUN-TO-DO EXERCISES FOR SPEEDY IMMUNE STIMULATION

First, select proper footwear and matting; you may do these to your favorite music.

AEROBIC DANCING—Select upbeat, catchy music for routines. Perform all exercises at a comfortable pace. Wear cushioned sneakers and use a well-cushioned floor mat.

STAIR-CLIMBING—Use handrails or wall for support. Walk up stairs at a comfortable pace. At top of stairs, turn around and descend forward. Wear cushioned sneakers. Go only one step at a time. Be careful to avoid any knee discomfort or steep steps.

SKIP-IN-PLACE—Place hands on hips and skip lightly on the balls of your feet. Legs should be at shoulder width and body weight should be shifted smoothly from one foot to the other.

JOG-IN-PLACE—Be sure to wear cushioned jogging shoes. Jog at a comfortable pace while landing on the balls of your feet. Bring knees up to waist level, with both arms pumping lightly. Your feet should always land in the same spot on the cushioned mat.

JUMPING JACKS—Stand with feet together and arms at side. Lightly jump up, bringing feet shoulder-width apart and both arms over head. Jump again, returning to original position and repeat.

ROPE SKIPPING—Use rope with a handle and make sure there's enough room for clearance. Skip lightly, landing on the balls of your feet. Avoid high-jumps.

The above exercises are simple and fun to do whenever you have free time. They are effective in alerting your sluggish immune system and building resistance to arthritis stiffness.

30 MINUTES OF EXERCISE A DAY KEEP ARTHRITIS AWAY

Telephone operator, Ruth B. D., had a sedentary job but there was no excuse for keeping in shape when she had spare time every evening and during weekends—and even during a long lunch hour.

So when she felt recurring painful spasms in her hips and lower back, she decided to nip the threat of arthritis in the bud with a fitness program. She devoted only 30 minutes daily to the aforedescribed easy exercises. Within two weeks, her stiffness and pains went away and she was more flexible than ever before. The simple exercises restored her range of motion to her hips and lower back. She continues them because "they're so much fun" and they also help keep arthritis away via a more stimulated immune system.

EXERCISE KEEPS YOUR NATURAL DEFENSE SYSTEM IN SHAPE

Your body has a natural defense system against arthritis invaders. A network of cells and substances will protect you against the invasion and spread of hurtful enemies. With the use of fitness, you will be able to revive your weakened defense system and keep your immune system strong enough to shield you from arthritic infection. Only *you* can use exercise for your immune system. Start right now!

IN REVIEW

1. Exercise is the key to a stronger immune system as well as pain control and healing of arthritis.
2. Strengthen your skeletal structure with regular exercise (as simple as a daily 30- to 60-minute brisk walk) so your immune system can make good use of nutritional barriers against arthritis.
3. Note the starting guidelines to help you fit exercise into your daily activities.
4. Jason R. M. overcame joint stiffness and inflammation with a simple set of nine range-of-motion exercises. It's fun to follow, too.
5. Enjoy a set of immune-invigorating exercises you can do anywhere in a matter of minutes.
6. Strengthen your bones with the easy exercises outlined.
7. Indoor exercises help speed immune stimulation against arthritis.

8. Ruth B. D. may have had a sedentary job that predisposed to hip and lower-back painful spasms, but 30 minutes of exercises daily helped keep arthritis away. You can do the same!

17

How to Protect Your Joints, Save Energy, and Resist Fatigue

Joint protection refers to doing everyday tasks, such as working and cleaning, in ways that reduce the stress on joints affected by arthritis. Overuse and abuse of joints with arthritis can further weaken your immune barrier. This may lead to pain and swelling, more joint damage, or loss of function and independence. You do need to keep active but within protective guidelines.

Inactivity Weakens the Immune System

When you become too sedentary, your immune system becomes sluggish and the important lymphocytes become weak and ineffective in guarding against hurtful invaders. This immune weakness because of inactivity causes muscles and bones to degenerate. Joints become ankylosed (stiff). Arthritis could take root and worsen.

White blood cells help your body fight infection. The type maintaining the front line of defense against arthritis enters your bloodstream *because of activity and exercise.* The white blood cells release a substance known as *pyrogen,* which stimulates body temperature to rise. When you are active, there is a healthy release of pyrogen which also boosts your body's immune response to ease arthritic discomfort.

Be cautious of inactivity which could result in chronic and oppressive degeneration of your joints and muscles.

Activity Is Good for You

Keeping active provides you with more energy, helps you sleep better, and also lessens stress. To understand, here is a thumbnail explanation about the structure of joints. A joint is the place in the body where two bones come together. Bone is living tissue that can grow and rebuild. Movement helps keep the bones strong. The ends of the bones are covered with cartilage. This is tough, elastic tissue that cushions and protects the bone ends. Easy, smooth activity is needed to nourish the cartilage.

Problem: If you do not move enough, your joints can become stiff. Your muscles become smaller and weaker. If you have a painful joint, you often keep it in a bent position because it feels better that way. However, if the joint stays bent too long it can become locked. The result can be deformity of that joint and loss of function.

Respect Pain: It's one of your body's signals that your immune system is weak. If you place your joints under harmful stress, you surely will feel pain. Do not take the attitude that you can "tough it out." If you overdo it today, you'll pay for it tomorrow! TIP: Be alert for pain that lasts for more than two hours after doing a task. If this happens, try doing the task differently the next time. Either use less effort or spend less time at it. (This applies to your exercise program as well.)

PROTECT YOURSELF AGAINST STRESS

Some positions and movements can put extra stress on joints. Even when these joints are not hot, swollen, and painful, they need to be used in their most stable postitions. *Avoid activities that involve a tight grip or that put too much pressure on your fingers.* If your hands are affected by arthritis, holding an object tightly can harm the already-damaged joints. Avoid twisting or using the joints forcefully. This also puts more stress on them. (See Figure 17–1.)

How to Open a Jar with Less Pain

Everyone has to open a screw-top jar from time to time. If you lean on the jar lid with the palm of your hand and turn the lid with a shoulder motion, you'll reduce stress to your fingers. You can make it easier still if you set the jar on a cloth on the counter or in the sink. You can also purchase a jar opener that allows you to hold the jar with two hands while turning it. You might also remind the family not to close jar lids too tightly the next time!

CONTROL YOUR WEIGHT

Extra pounds put even more stress on *weight-bearing joints* (hips, knees, back, and feet). This extra stress can lead to further joint pain and damage. If you are overweight, lose some of those extra pounds. Your immune system functions better. You'll also look better, have more energy, and feel healthier, too.

AVOID HOLDING ONE POSITION FOR A LONG TIME

If you keep joints or muscles in the same position for a long time, you could increase pain and stiffness. *Example:* Writing a long letter keeps your hand in the same position for as long as it takes time to finish the letter. TIP: Relax and stretch your hand and arm every five minutes or so.

USE YOUR STRONGEST JOINTS AND MUSCLES

Remember to use the strongest joints and muscles whenever possible. Here are some examples:

*Carry a purse over your shoulder on a strap, rather than holding it in your hand.

*Push open a heavy door with the side of your arm, not with your hand and outstretched arm.

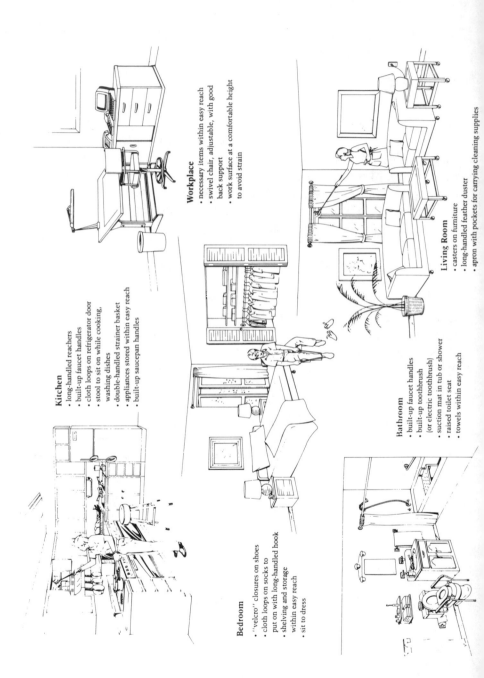

Kitchen
- long-handled reachers
- built-up faucet handles
- cloth loops on refrigerator door
- stool to sit on while cooking, washing dishes
- double-handled strainer basket
- appliances stored within easy reach
- built-up saucepan handles

Workplace
- necessary items within easy reach
- swivel chair, adjustable, with good back support
- work surface at a comfortable height to avoid strain

Bedroom
- "velcro" closures on shoes
- cloth loops on socks to put on with long-handled hook
- shelving and storage within easy reach
- sit to dress

Bathroom
- built-up faucet handles
- built-up toothbrush (or electric toothbrush)
- suction mat in tub or shower
- raised toilet seat
- towels within easy reach

Living Room
- casters on furniture
- long-handled feather duster
- apron with pockets for carrying cleaning supplies

Figure 17-1

*When using stairs, lead with your stronger leg going *up* and your weaker leg going *down.*

*When lifting something that is low or on the ground, bend your knees and lift with your back straight.

*To get up from a chair, slide forward with knees together, feet flat on the floor, and tucked in close to the chair. Lean slightly forward. Push down with your palms on the arm of the chair (or the seat if there are no arms.) Push up with your hips and knees.

*Remember, also, to spread the weight of an object over many joints to reduce the stress placed on one joint.

*Use the palms of both hands to lift and hold cups, plates, pots, or pans rather than gripping them with your fingers or one hand only. Use padded oven mitts for hot dishes.

*Carry heavy loads in your arms instead of gripping them with your fingers or hands.

*Spread your hand flat over a sponge or rag instead of squeezing it with your fingers.

BALANCE REST AND ACTIVITY

Take short rest periods throughout the day. Learn to balance periods of work with rest breaks so that you do not place too much stress on your joints or get too tired.

While on the job, change positions and stretch your muscles often to avoid stiffness. Take short breaks. Alternate activities throughout the day.

If you wash and wax your car and find that your joints hurt two hours after you've finished, then you have overdone it. Next time, take a break between washing and waxing and another one before you polish.

If you enjoy yard work, use long-handled tools or a gardening stool designed to reduce the stress on your back and legs. Specially made, lightweight gardening tools can reduce joint stress. Avoid any activity that puts a strain on joints where you have pain or stiffness. For example, if your wrist is sore, you shouldn't play tennis. However, you might be able to swim instead.

Of course, the kind of activity, how much time you spend on it, and the length and number of your rest breaks will probably change from day to day. You will soon learn to balance rest and activity according to how you feel.

PACE YOURSELF FOR MORE ENERGY

Pace yourself not only during the day but also from day to day. Allow plenty of time to finish the things you start, so you will not feel rushed. Don't try to do too much at one time.

Suggestion: Each night, prepare a written schedule of the next day's tasks. Think about what they involve—the amount of time they require and how tiring they are. Be realistic. Scheduling and pacing also include doing the hardest things when you're feeling your best.

Balancing rest and activity may seem like a juggling act, but soon enough you will discover that it *can* be done. As any juggler knows, the fewer things you are trying to balance, the easier it is to do!

ORGANIZE WORK AND STORAGE AREAS

In your work area, keep all the equipment necessary for any task together in one area. For example, for baking, keep your mixing bowls, sifter, measuring cups, and spoons in one place. As a general rule, try to put those items you use most often nearest your work area and less-used items farther away.

Organize your cleaning supplies so they are easy to reach and easy to replace when you're finished using them. Keep the same cleaning supplies in several places: kitchen and bathroom, upstairs and downstairs.

SIT TO WORK

If possible, sit to work at a comfortable height. Don't strain your shoulders or neck. Try to take the weight off your hips, knees, and ankles. Many tasks you do standing can be done seated. For example, sit to cook, iron, wash dishes, and even to dress. A high stool may be useful for some of these tasks.

ON THE JOB

A well-designed chair should provide good back support, and should swivel or be easily moved. It also should be adjustable to the proper height for any activity.

Work surfaces (whether you sit or stand) should be at a height so your elbows are at right angles and your shoulders are relaxed when you work. If you work at a desk, a slanted top (or a drafting table) will raise the material, reducing the strain on your neck and upper back. If you use tools, place them at a convenient level. Build up the handles to avoid a tight grasp.

If your job requires that you stand, your work surface should be at a comfortable height. Take frequent rest periods—try to lie down for a while or sit if lying is not possible. While working, shift your weight from one leg to the other by placing one foot on a step or stool in front of you.

CUSHIONS PAIN WITH SIMPLE ADJUSTMENTS IN ACTIVITIES

When the alarm clock went off, Barbara DeG. was ready to throw a pillow at it but her arthritis limited her range of motion. All she could do was fret and fume because she faced a day filled with pain because daily activities caused excessive joint abuse. Shutting off the alarm, she struggled to get out of bed and took "forever" to get started for her part-time job. It, too, was hurtful to her already aching joints. She felt if her movements were further restricted, she might become an invalid. A co-worker who faced the same immune deficiency problem of arthritic flareup was able to move around with greater ease. The secret?

She told Barbara DeG. that her chiropractor outlined simple suggestions for getting through the day at work and at home. The suggestions included do-it-yourself protection guidelines as outlined above. Barbara DeG. followed the methods and before too long, she was so relieved, she could throw a pillow at the alarm clock (only to prove to herself that she could do it!) and bounce out of bed, eager to face a pain-reduced workday.

USE LABOR-SAVING ITEMS

Try to avoid bending, stooping, and reaching as much as possible. Use labor-saving devices. These are available in local hardware and variety stores, pharmacies, health stores, and medical supply shops.

For example, you can use equipment with enlarged handles. Build up the handles on pens, eating utensils, tools, brushes, and any other objects you use often.

Tape a layer or two of thin foam rubber around the handles (or use a foam rubber hair curler). Use long-handled tongs to reach objects on a high shelf or on the floor. Electric appliances, such as can openers, blenders, knives, and scissors get the job done with less time and energy.

You might also consider using a wheeled cart to move heavy things from place to place in the kitchen or from room to room (such as laundry after it's been washed and dried.)

Make things easier for your joints but not to the point where you become inactive since this could create a sluggish immune system and a more serious arthritis invasion.

REFUSES TO TAKE ARTHRITIS "LYING DOWN"

When Philip R. R. developed painful knees, he avoided using them, spending long periods in front of the television set with his legs propped up. This inactivity caused a weakness in his immune system which only made his arthritis worse. Because he developed night-time leg cramps, he sought medical help and only routinely told the general practitioner about his arthritic knees.

The doctor told him to "get up and start moving," but without strain to the joints. "If you let arthritis spread by lying down, you face the possibility of becoming an invalid. You *can* recharge your immune system to cast out hurtful invaders if you keep yourself active . . . within reason, of course."

Philip R. R. rearranged his residential and working conditions with some of the preceding labor-saving (but not labor-ending) methods. The knee pains slowly subsided; night leg pains vanished speedily. By refusing to take arthritis "lying down," he was soon flexible and energetic with minimal symptoms.

The outcome of arthritis depends not only on the process of the condition, but also on your personal methods of coping with it. It is important to practice joint protection and also to keep yourself active. With these aids, you can help your immune system keep arthritis away at arm's length—and a straight pain-free arm at that!

IN REVIEW

1. Supercharge your immune system with activity to help cast out arthritis invaders. Strain, but not to the point of pain, for good results!

2. Rearrange your lifestyle to accommodate any limitations. Use your strongest joints and muscles. Make things easier for yourself to conserve energy and protect against fatigue.

3. Whether at work or at home, some simple rearrangements will help protect your joints and enable you to get things done without pain.

4. Barbara DeG. used simple suggestions to protect her abused joints and was soon able to move with a pain-reduced flexibility.

5. Philip R. R. recharged his immune system by getting up from his couch, keeping active, and using labor-saving methods. His knee-pains and night leg-pains vanished speedily.

18

Free Yourself from Pain Without Drugs

Pain is a symptom—a warning signal telling your body to fight against the invasion of irritants, or prepare for current or impending injury. Pain is generally classified into two types:

(1) *Acute pain,* such as that following injury or surgery; it can be mild to severe and is of limited duration. It is a sensation triggered in the nervous system to alert you to possible injury and to take better care of yourself.

(2) *Chronic pain,* such as headaches and backaches that can last for weeks, months, or even years. It can be disabling. It is all-too-familiar in arthritis which has recurring pain over a long period of time.

Pain and Emotions

For many, pain is worse at night. In the dark and the quiet, when we're alone with our thoughts, we concentrate more on our pain. What had been mild often turns severe. Pain's intensity is often affected by your overall condition and mental attitude. Bump your head one day and you think nothing of it. Do it again weeks later, after you've had a dispute with someone or if you're depressed, and the pain could be much more intense.

CHARTING THE PATHWAY OF PAIN

Invaders penetrating the immune system are responsible for pain. To understand this pathway, it is helpful to scan your immune system and thereby come up with drug-free boosting methods.

How the Immune System Protects Against Pain

The process begins with the macrophage, a scavenger cell. Its task is to move throughout your body, locate damaged cells or foreign invaders such as a virus, and ingest them. During this digestion and self-cleansing process, the macrophage places fragments of the cell's proteins into a number of HLA molecules which lie on the surface of every macrophage. This process informs your immune system about the presence of these fragments and materials.

If your immune system, beginning with the T-cells, "sees" the materials as being "alien" to your body (if it is a virus, for instance), then your immune system rises up to destroy the virus. If the ingested cell was a "self"-cell (taken from your own body), the T-cells read this and your immune system is not activated.

Problem: If you have an autoimmune illness such as arthritis, there is a miscommunication between T-cells and HLA molecules. Even though no "alien" material is in your body, your immune system still becomes activated. It springs into battle and attacks selected groups of your body's own healthy cells. This is an autoimmune misfire. The symptoms and arthritis condition is the result of an interaction of complex factors.

The number of HLA molecules can increase dramatically during an infectious attack. As an autoimmune disease, arthritis may result from an unfortunate convergence of any such factors—a certain T-cell coming in contact with a large number of certain HLA molecules; a higher-than-normal concentration of "self"-proteins in one area; a gathering of "self"-proteins in an area of the body where they are not normally seen; a coincidental increase of "self"-proteins in one area *and* an unusual number of HLA molecules on the surfaces of scavenger cells. Any or all of these situations tend to deceive the immune system, present it with something unusual. The immune system attacks and you feel pain!

During this pain attack, cells of the injured tissue release histamine, prostaglandin, and bradykinin which irritate local nerve endings and dispatch pain messages toward your brain. The hurt nerve endings send an electrochemical impulse through the nerves to your spinal cord, through which nerve signals from all parts of the body must pass en route to the brain. From the spinal cord, the impulse moves up to the thalamus region of the brain and to the cerebral cortex. All this information is then sent back down the pain pathways, while further information ascends. This is felt as arthritic hurt, acute or chronic. (See Figure 18–1.)

UPWARD PAIN SIGNALS

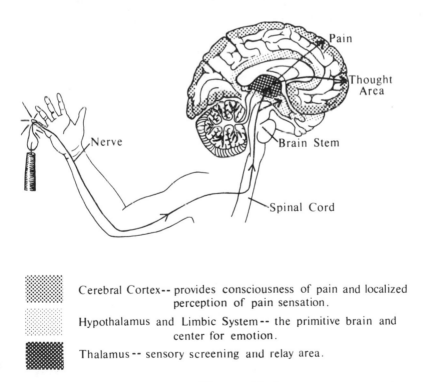

Cerebral Cortex-- provides consciousness of pain and localized perception of pain sensation.

Hypothalamus and Limbic System-- the primitive brain and center for emotion.

Thalamus-- sensory screening and relay area.

ILLUSTRATION—THE UPJOHN COMPANY

Figure 18–1

ENDORPHINS: YOUR BODY'S NATURAL PAIN KILLERS

Your immune system is able to manufacture its own *natural* pain killer. Within your brain are special "receptors" for these natural substances. Receptors are chemical structures often located on the surfaces of cells that serve as reception points for body-made substances and drugs. Each type of receptor is like a lock that can be turned only by a certain key. Your immune system is that key!

To ease arthritic pain, your immune system alerts your brain to set off the release of an important pain killer—the family of *endorphins*. These are immune-stimulated compounds with morphine-like properties, such as the ability to change pain perception, mood, respiration rate, and release of certain hormones. Endorphins have been found in many parts of the body, but are concentrated mostly in the brain and spinal cord, particularly in areas concerned with the transmission of pain signals.

Endorphins are able to block the pain-causing effects of histamine, prostaglandin, and bradykinin which are involved in arthritis hurt and discomfort. Immunologists observe that to relieve arthritis, an endorphin-releasing pain-killer is needed. It is available through (1) drugs and (2) natural stimulation of the immune system. Which method should you consider?

PAIN KILLERS CAN GIVE YOU A PAIN

Drugs are potent weapons in the battle against arthritis pain. But they are not panaceas. They are not miracles in a capsule. Every drug has adverse side effects. Many analgesics, as pain-killers are called, are narcotic, and physical/mental addiction may result from extended use. More familiar are side effects from common and uncommon "everyday" drugs that play havoc with an already abused and weakened immune system:

Aspirin. Non-narcotic and mild. Reduces fever and pain. *Side Effects:* Ringing in ears; hearing loss may occur with intake of 6 grams per day. Dizziness, vomiting, sweating, flushing, fever, hyperventilation, gastric irritation, drowsiness.

Acetaminophen. Non-narcotic and mild. Reduces fever, inflammation and pain. *Side Effects:* Liver problems, toxicity, nausea, vomiting, loss of appetite, sweating, possible abdominal pain with enlargement of liver and spleen.

Ibuprofen. Non-narcotic and more powerful. A non-steroid anti-inflammatory drug that eases inflammation. *Side Effects:* May have dependency reaction, nausea, vomiting, or drowsiness.

Codeine. Narcotic and mild. Eases pain. *Side Effects:* Nausea, constipation, dizziness, flushed face, fatigue, dulls alertness and reflexes. Prescription drug.

Propoxyphene. Narcotic and mild. Eases pain. Similar to codeine. *Side Effects:* Stomach upset; mild risk of nausea and constipation. Prescription drug.

Meperidine. Narcotic, strong. Soothes pain. *Side Effects:* Nausea, digestive upset. Potentially very addictive. Prescription drug.

Hydromorphone. Narcotic, very strong. Eases pain. Similar to codeine. *Side Effects:* Produces a powerful high. Reactions are accentuated when dosages are boosted to maintain initial high and pain-killing effect. Vomiting and loss of mental alertness is likely to occur. Potentially very addictive. Prescription drug.

Morphine. Narcotic, very strong. Eases pain. *Side Effects:* Could lead to nausea and loss of mental alertness. Potentially very addictive. Prescription drug.

Drugs Abuse Immune System

Drugs create reactions that abuse and hurt an already weakened immune system, and this causes a "circle" in which the pain and inflammation may be eased—but constant narcotics, whether prescribed or not, will further lower your pain threshold. Since most drugs become tolerated by the body necessitating increased dosages, it becomes a threat to your immune system as time goes on. You go around and around, and, in the end, your hurt remains (perhaps worse) and your drugs are constantly being increased and changed. What is the answer to living without pain and without drugs?

Stimulate Your Immune System

Modalities are available to stimulate your immune system via your brain receptors to release a sufficient amount of endorphins to create a form of natural pain relief.

Endorphins join with *enkephalins,* another naturally produced chemical that has a morphine-like action. Together, they act as your body's own opiates. They can provide relief from arthritis pain and inflammation. Your option: Instead of reaching for a drug . . . reach for a natural method to stimulate your own pain-relieving reaction.

WILLOW BARK—"NATURAL ASPIRIN"

Aspirin in its natural form is obtained from the bark of the willow tree and was first prescribed more than 2,000 years ago by Hippocrates, the ancient Greek father of medicine.

"Natural Aspirin" Soothes Arthritic Pain

Willow bark is available through herbalists and herbal pharmacies. It works to inhibit your body's production of prostaglandins, the hormone-like substances produced in response to immune invaders. Willow bark will help interfere with the production of various PGs, as they are called, and stimulate your immune system to alert your macrophages and your HLA molecules to uproot and cast out virus invaders.

Eases Inflammation

During arthritic inflammation, white blood cells rush to the troubled area to consume toxic materials and debris. There is also an increase in the circulation of body fluids to wash away accumulated wastes. This increased activity and fluid account for the warmth, swelling, redness, and pain of your inflammation. Prostaglandins trigger inflammation. Willow bark has a PG-fighting activity that alerts your immune system to protect against painful swelling and reduce inflammation. You enjoy freedom from arthritis hurt and inflammation—without the risk of narcotic addiction or side effects.

HERBAL REMEDIES TO BUILD IMMUNITY TO ARTHRITIC PAIN

For soothing of pain and/or inflammation, consider alternatives to chemical dependency with herbal home remedies.

Black Birch Salve—Mix some of the sap from the black birch tree with a bit of Vaseline. Massage afflicted joints with it, rubbing in as much as possible. Apply a thin coating for daytime wear. Repeat morning and night.

Burdock Tea—Brew a tea of burdock roots or leaves and sip slowly for relief of discomfort.

Pokeberries—Eat fresh or dried pokeberries to help soothe pain. Start with a few daily and gradually increase the amount.

Solomon's Seal Tea—Brew a tea and sip slowly with a bit of lemon juice and honey, if desired. Helps protect against pain flareups.

Starweed Leaves—Soak the leaves of starweed in water and apply to the affected area for speedy relief and comfort.

Willow Bark Tea—Sip the tea regularly to help strengthen your immune system and resist painful reactions.

Yarrow Herb Tea—A flavorful tea that herbalists prescribe to ease joint stiffness and pain.

Wintergreen Oil Liniment—A prime source of natural methyl salicylate which helps provide a soothing, penetrating benefit by easing spasms and wincing pain.

Herbal remedies ranging from willow bark (the "natural aspirin") to yarrow herb tea are to be considered in your search for a drugless means of helping your immune system cast out arthritis!

ENJOYS FREEDOM FROM PAIN WITH "NATURAL ASPIRIN"

Shooting spasms of pain and frequent bouts with inflammation made Katy O'L. so desperate, she would take any available drug that promised relief. Yes, she had some merciful easing of symptoms, but her body tolerated drugs and she had to take increasingly higher dosages. She also paid the penalty with side effects including embarrassing nausea, insomnia, and gastro-intestinal upset.

She felt she was in a tight squeeze. If she gave up aspirin, she would have recurring pains and inflammation. If she took the drug, she had a tradeoff in terms of reduced arthritis but increased side effects. Katy O'L. sought help from a recommended herbal pharmacist. He suggested she take willow bark capsules in doses recommended by her health practitioner. Katy O'L. gave up drugs for three days to try this "natural aspirin."

Almost within hours, the willow bark ingredients worked to block hurtful PGs and also strengthened her immune system to ease inflammatory discomfort. By the end of the third day, she told her smiling herbal pharmacist she would now rely exclusively on the willow bark because it worked fast and she was not only free of her arthritis pain . . . but also free of the dangerous side effects of drugs.

THE AMINO ACID THAT "CHASES AWAY" ARTHRITIS PAIN

An essential amino acid, L-tryptophan has an analgesic action (pain-relieving) which boosts the immune system to release gamma-interferon and interleuken-2, which strengthen the body's resistance against invaders.

L-tryptophan works best when taken with Vitamin B3 (niacin) and B6 (pyridoxine). It is converted in your brain to serotonin, a neurotransmitter that produces a feeling of relaxation, serenity, and even freedom from depression.

L-tryptophan strengthens the power of your immune system to "chase away" hurtful invaders to blame for arthritic pain. It further benefits with its ability to bring about a comfortable sleep and ease stress. (Insomnia and tension are obviously involved in the causes of pain.)

Taking L-Tryptophan

Official requirements call for 3 milligrams daily for every 2.2 pounds of adult body weight. You may need more if you are a chronic pain victim. For example, a healthy 150-pounder requires only 200 milligrams daily. But the pain-filled arthritic of the same weight requires 3,000 or more to help the immune system "surround and deport" pain invaders!

Food Sources of L-Tryptophan

Eggs, 2 large	422 milligrams
Peanuts, shelled, ¾ cup	367 milligrams
Peanut butter, 6 tablespoons	336 milligrams
Liver, calf's, 3 ounces, cooked	292 milligrams
Chicken, fryer, 3 ounces	286 milligrams
Cheddar cheese, 3 ounces	270 milligrams
Beef, round, 3 ounces	260 milligrams
Halibut, 3 ounces	211 milligrams

Additional sources of L-tryptophan would be most meats, seafood, poultry, cheese, dairy products, and soybeans. From the above, it would seem difficult to have at least 3,000 milligrams daily from food. Most of the preceding may be nourishing but also contain cholesterol, fat, calories, and sodium which is unwise for the arthritic immune system.

Simple Daily L-Tryptophan Plan

Include moderate amounts of the preceding L-tryptophan foods in your daily meal program. *Supplements:* Discuss potency with your health practitioner. Most have found a revitalization of the immune system on 3,000 to 4,000 milligrams daily. A rule-of-thumb is to start by taking 500 milligrams four or five times daily, at meals and bedtime.

After one week, increase bedtime potency to 1,000 or 1,500 milligrams. Most have reported finding relief after three weeks and can gradually reduce L-tryptophan dosage to about 1,500 to 2,000 milligrams daily for comfort and freedom from symptoms.

Be on the Lookout: You may have some reactions such as fatigue, nasal congestion, and a respiratory blockage. This is evidence your immune system is boosting your interferon and interleuken-2 defenders to cleanse your body of invaders. Best to ease up on potency and reduce L-tryptophan dosage until these so-called "side effects" go away. Very few have told of these reactions, though.

Important: L-tryptophan cannot be converted into the neurotransmitter serotonin without sufficient amounts of Vitamin B3 (niacin) and B6 (pyridoxine), so aim for a balanced intake.

SIMPLE NUTRIENT HEALS "LIFELONG" PAIN

Lester LaJ. experienced worsening pains, especially in his back and hip region with recurring flareups of inflammation that made it difficult to move his joints when sitting or trying to stand up. It was agonizing to get in and out of a car. Elbow joint pains soon spread until his wrists and fingers became hurtfully inflamed and swollen. As a tool and die mechanic, his means of livelihood was in jeopardy. He tried the wide range of prescribed and over-the-counter drugs. They had minimal effect. He feared becoming addicted to stronger dosages of narcotics. Was there any alternative?

A co-worker told Lester LaJ. of an orthopedist who outlined a nutritional program that restored the immune system of his relative and eliminated the pain and inflammation. Lester LaJ. appeared for a diagnosis and told of his disdain for drugs. He was given a program that called for L-tryptophan along with niacin and pyridoxine. This three-pronged program worked within days. His back and hips became free of painful spasms. He had restored flexibility. His elbow, wrists, and fingers soon became so revitalized, he could work with the greatest of ease. He had restored the full power of his immune system so that the pain-causing, inflammation-producing invaders were seized and destroyed and his resistance restored. All this . . . without harmful drugs!

BIOFEEDBACK IS HELPFUL IN MANY SITUATIONS

Biofeedback is a form of meditation hooked up to a monitoring device. As one or another of your body's indicators of stress reverses toward normal, the monitoring device flashes or buzzes or swings its meter dial or even plays triumphant music. It is a helpful device if your pain is stress-produced.

For example, by using the biofeedback machine, you can become aware that a particular event, mood, thought, or person makes you tense (tension does contribute to arthritic spasms and pain because of a weakness in the immune system), and then you can learn to avoid it.

How Does Biofeedback Work?

Some believe that pain is controlled by or minimized because of a distraction element, or because the arthritic has a sense of control over the pain; there could be a hypnotic-like suggestion from the biofeedback operator. One belief is that biofeedback acts as a teaching mechanism, showing a person on a ticker tape or graph what is happening inside the body at the moment it happens. The arthritic may then be able to guard against a particular action that is causing the pain; you learn how to manipulate the pain by manipulating the graph.

For example, if the biofeedback's electrodes are placed on your wrists and if you clench your fingers, you will see a rise in the tension of your muscles, graphically represented by a meter.

Therefore, if electrodes are attached to a point where you feel pain, and you watch that pain (as muscle tension) register on the graph, you should be able to reduce your discomfort (if tension-caused) by making a strong emotional effort to relax. While watching the biofeedback display screen, you can use different relaxation methods until you see the meter reading drop which simultaneously means a drop in pain.

Emotions, Immune System, Self-Healing

Emotions do stimulate your brain receptors to release endorphins and enkephalins, valuable pain-killers needed by your immune system to "dilute" and "defuse" the hurt of histamine, prostaglandin, and bradykinin in your system. Some immunologists feel a certain amount of self-healing is possible if you have a "mental calm" that will reduce pain and spasms. When you are able to gain control over your body and its responses, your "mental calm" may well be able to supercharge your immune system with pain-killing endorphins.

Biofeedback may be of help in this immune rebuilding purpose. Such machines are available for home use. But you may want to try a simple, "do-it-yourself" biofeedback remedy without the machine.

Biofeedback at Home Without the Machine

Are you all wrought up with stress or tension? Simple biofeedback techniques are: monitor your own pulse—and if it is excessively rapid, you are tense; use a mirror to observe the tightening of facial muscles; try a ring thermometer which is easy to read and see if you are being troubled with heavy blood surges. The point is to *know* when you are tense and how to control the situation. Biofeedback helps you accept total relaxation techniques as natural remedies. Once you use these total relaxation techniques as part of your pain control, immune-building program, you may no longer need biofeedback. You need to restore complete confidence that your mind *can* help you control arthritic pain via a stronger immune system.

PAIN, IMMUNE SYSTEM, ARTHRITIS

Your body organs have many fine nerve fibers called *nociceptors,* which are sensitive to intense, potentially harmful hurt. When an injury occurs, your immune system is galvanized into action. There is a release of the pain-causing chemicals (histamine, prostaglandins, bradykinin) which lower your body's *pain threshold* (the level at which a sensation becomes painful). You then become more sensitive to arthritis which is linked to hurtful prostaglandin production. The pain message shoots from the injured area, to the spinal cord, then to the brain.

Your body can reduce pain through use of nutritional and natural therapies which alert your *opiate receptors* on the surface of your neurons (nerve cells). An outpouring of endorphins ("the morphine within") creates a healing reaction. All this happens when you supercharge your immune system with home-based, practical "natural medicines."

IN REVIEW

1. Chart the pathway of pain. Help your body release healing endorphins.
2. Pain killers can give you a pain! Seek natural substitutes for drugs.

3. Katy O'L. used willow bark as a "natural aspirin" and recovered from arthritis without any of the frightening drug side effects.

4. Boost immune function with herbal remedies and L-tryptophan, the amino acid that "chases away" arthritic pain.

5. Lester LaJ. followed a simple nutritional program that healed "lifelong" pain without the use of narcotic drugs.

6. Biofeedback can easily be followed at home without complicated machinery to help you predict and prevent pain with "mental calm."

19

Your Immune-Building Food Program to Heal Arthritis

Foods have the ability to revive your weakened natural defense system to uproot and cast out arthritic invaders. To restore your immune system to optimal performance, plan your nutritional program around specific nutrients and foods. Your goal is to arm your immune system to fight viral enemies and guard against arthritic pain and invasion. Important nutrients include:

Vitamin A. Helps maintain the number of T-cells, the immune-building attack soldiers who knock out viral enemies. Helps maintain cell maturity, preventing cells from reverting back to immature forms that are characteristic of arthritis. Also acts as an antioxidant to help in protecting against malignant cells.

Vitamin B-Complex. Particularly B6, and also pantothenic and folic acids, which are needed to make the crucial virus-fighting antibodies. They stimulate the immune system, participate in biological reactions that produce immune cells and have a direct deleterious effect on arthritis cells.

241

Vitamin C. Inhibits virus intrusion into the cells. Essential in the formation of white blood cells—your immune system's "hit men"; helps ease stress; protects your circulatory system from clogging fat deposits; and strengthens connective tissue between the cells. Vitamin C is a necessary component in the process that produces an enzyme, C1 esterase, needed by your immune system to recognize foreign invaders in the body. Without this enzyme, arthritis cells would go undetected and they could seize hold of your body. Vitamin C also increases the number of lymphocytes in the blood. The vitamin initiates the genesis of lymphoblasts—the immature bone marrow and lymph gland cells that create lymphocytes. Vitamin C works with zinc, linoleic acid, and Vitamin B6 (pyridoxine) to produce T-lymphocytes. It is also believed that Vitamin C boosts activity of interferon, your body's built-in virus-fighting substance.

Zinc. Vital for boosting the immune system. Needed to invigorate your lymph system, especially the thymus gland where important T-cells develop. The concentration of zinc in your cells determines how energetically antibodies attack arthritis invaders.

Enzymes. Found only in fresh, raw fruits and vegetables and their juices. Cooking and processing will destroy enzyme content. Enzymes are catalysts—speeding up reactions in the body. Enzymes are spark-plugs. They invigorate the action of natural defense cells and their antibodies.

While all vitamins and minerals and other nutrients are needed to build and sustain a strong immune system, the preceding elements appear to be in the spotlight in your arthritis-healing program.

A DOCTOR'S DIET PLAN TO HELP YOU FIGHT BACK AGAINST ARTHRITIS

To improve or recover from arthritis, your body is helped with proper nutrition as a cornerstone of therapy. "Arthritis does not come on overnight and no change in the diet will work an overnight 'cure.' However, the proper combination of the best 'body-building' foods and the elimination of the allergic and low quality foods will improve health and help you fight back against arthritis," says Robert Bingham, M.D., of the Desert Arthritis Medical Clinic in Desert Hot Springs, California.

Importance of Nutrition

"Arthritis is treatable. It can be arrested and is often curable. Most arthritis patients do not know that nutrition is such an important factor in the cause and treatment of their disease. They are often satisfied with the quality of their dietary intake. *But good nutrition and the correction of dietary deficiencies is necessary for the successful treatment of all types of arthritis.*

"Some types of arthritis can be relieved or 'cured' by therapeutic nutrition alone, but therapy for rheumatoid and osteoarthritis must include correction of metabolic as well as nutritional deficiencies.

"When the physician is not educated in the value of good nutrition, then *the patient must take the initiative to learn his own personal needs and to supply them.* The use of applied nutrition in the treatment of arthritis differs from the usual medical treatment routines in that it will produce improvement and even recovery in many early cases."

Dr. Bingham, who has healed thousands of patients at his clinic over three decades, offers this immune-boosting diet program:

Foods Should Be Fresh

Processing, over-refining, and additives destroy many nutrients and may introduce undesirable and harmful chemicals. Take care against overcooking and too-high temperatures which destroy nutrients. Select foods that are raw, fresh, and naturally grown as much as possible. Frozen foods may have lost some food value but are preferred over canned and packaged foods. Oils, salad dressings, butter, etc., should be refrigerated to protect against rancidity, which (however slight) destroys many nutrients and may create arthritic reactions in some sensitive people.

Carbohydrates for Immune Energy

Natural, unrefined carbohydrates are available in whole grains, fresh fruits, and vegetables and also cooked legumes. They regulate protein and fat metabolism and function as a major energy source for immune-related metabolic functions.

Fats Are Needed for Metabolic Functions

In particular, linoleic, linolenic, and arachidonic acids (not produced by the body) are needed to break down clogging cholesterol and saturated fats. Unrefined oils are needed from nuts, grains, and vegetables. Safflower (linoleic), soy (linolenic), and peanut (arachidonic) oils are highest in essential fatty acids. Other good sources are sunflower, sesame, walnut, corn, and olive oils. Your fats should come largely from vegetable sources in moderate amounts. A little goes a long way. Avoid heated fats whenever possible.

Fiber Scrubs Away Debris

Select a variety of high-fiber foods rather than only one or two sources. Fiber is found in whole grains, nuts, legumes, fruits, and vegetables. Fiber helps cleanse the body of damaged and unclean cells to allow your immune system to function at full force.

Meat May Be Used

Meats are good sources of the B-complex vitamins, iron, trace minerals, and protein. Eat meat once a week, preferably at breakfast—"unless sufficient proteins are supplied from other sources," says Dr. Bingham. Remove visible fat. Choose fresh or frozen meats rather than canned (except for tuna and salmon). Guard against processed or packaged meats (hot dogs, lunchmeats, salami, etc.) which contain fat and chemicals and should be avoided entirely.

Fruits and Vegetables

They should be fresh, naturally grown, and superior in food value to frozen or canned produce, especially when eaten raw. Naturally ripened or sun-dried fruits, along with citrus fruits and juices with pulp, are rich in vitamins, minerals, and enzymes.

Grains and Nuts

Fresh, stoneground cereals and flours supply vitamins, iron, and some protein and minerals. But bread is the "staff of life" only when it is made from the whole grain and contains the vitamins and trace minerals found in the germ, or berry, of the grain. Choose only *wholegrain* products: brown rice, whole wheat and rye, yellow corn meal, buckwheat, millet, oats, or freshly milled wheat germ. Bran or wheat germ may be added to other cereals, pancakes, waffles, muffins, etc. Granola is the best cold cereal. Nuts and seeds should be whole, fresh, and unsalted. Try sunflower, pumpkin, sesame seeds, almonds, walnuts, etc. Nut butters should be non-hydrogenated and without additives. To obtain a lower fat content, pour off excess oil from the top. Avoid cracked nuts or broken pieces which are often rancid. Avoid foods made from enriched, refined flour.

Dairy Products

Milk is essential for all ages. Two or three glasses daily (or equivalent in buttermilk, cottage cheese, yogurt) provide many nutrients. Certified raw milk, if available, is highly recommended. "It is especially valuable for those with a tendency to arthritis," says Dr. Bingham, "because it is higher in enzymes, growth factors, Wulzen factors, protein, minerals, fats, and natural vitamins than pasteurized milk." Buttermilk has the same protein value as whole milk and contains no more fat than skim milk. Yogurt goes well with fruit and in salads; it is essential in high-protein and low-fat reducing diets. Cottage cheese is a good base for salads. Natural, unprocessed cheeses are great sources of protein and far more nutritious than processed, chemicalized cheeses, spreads, and margarine. Skim milk cheese is a suitable alternative. (NOTE: The Wulzen Factor is an anti-stiffness substance found in raw milk; the factor is destroyed in pasteurization.)

Beverages

Coffee and tea are *not* recommended beverages. Excessive consumption may cause facial rash or chest pains. Caffeine-free beverages may be used but do not sweeten. Avoid soft drinks because of their sugar, caffeine, and chemical content. Alcohol should be restricted because of the damage it does to tissues. Choose caffeine-free herbal teas and coffee substitutes, if you must.

Desserts

Fruits, cheese, simple puddings, and custards are best for desserts. Use honey and maple sugar with discretion. Avoid white sugar in any form. Chocolate contains oxalates which interfere with calcium absorption. Carob is an acceptable substitute for chocolate-like flavor but is higher in fat content.

Spices

Use a variety of herbs and spices in cooking for flavoring: thyme, rosemary, sage, cinnamon, etc. They add food interest and stimulate the appetite and gastric juices. Watch labels for hidden salts in foods.

Dr. Bingham points out, "Nutrients should *not* be considered as medicinal agents since they function in an entirely different way. Medicines and drugs interfere with metabolism, but nutrients make metabolism possible. They are the raw materials from which metabolic machinery is built. Life cannot exist without them."[1]

RELIEVES PAIN AND BOOSTS IMMUNITY TO ARTHRITIS

Textile salesman Clifford D. N. was troubled with a weak immune system traced to stress caused by constant travel. Eating at fast-food outlets led to nutritional deficiencies and fat overload. Frequent painful spasms, especially upon awakening, brought him to a nutrition-aware internist. A thorough exam showed a weakened defense system that allowed penetration of harmful viral agents. He outlined a nutritional program based upon Dr. Robert Bingham's discoveries. Within four weeks, Clifford D. N. was free of pain and favored with an anti-arthritis immune system!

---

[1] Robert Bingham, M.D., Desert Hot Springs, California, personal communication.

FOUR FOODS THAT HELP BUILD IMMUNE RESISTANCE TO ARTHRITIS

A balance of healthful foods will help strengthen your immune system, yet specific foods may often have unusual abilities to promote production of arthritis-fighting antibodies. Plan to use them in your meal program as frequently as possible.

GARLIC. This potent vegetable more than doubles the potency of your natural killer T-cells, those powerful lymphocytes that destroy arthritis cells but leave the normal ones unharmed. Garlic contains allicin, a key anti-bacterial and anti-viral substance. Several garlic cloves daily—especially raw and in a fresh salad—will help pass into your digestive system and then into your bloodstream where they could kill the free-floating viruses. The power of garlic is that it may kill the viruses within your cells and thereby build immunity to arthritis and other conditions.

ONION. A relative of garlic so its benefits enhance the immune situation. An anti-thrombatic factor inhibits blood clots. In its complex organic structure, the onion bulb develops a molecular substance of sulfuric acid known as allinin. This is a powerful antibiotic and antibacterial reaction that will help boost the immune system.

FIGS. A prime source of calcium and fiber, and also a score of nutrients needed to boost the immune system. A natural sweet, too. Figs contain a protein-dissolving enzyme called *ficin* or *cradein* which will help to destroy harmful invaders in the cells. Its bulk fiber and seeds also correct constipation.

PAPAYA. Contains *papain,* an enzyme capable of digesting tough protein and fats, too. To help protect your cells from fatty overload, include Hawaiian papaya as a dessert in your meal plans. It will help cleanse your cells of debris and allow immune-releasing T-cells to move swiftly through your body to cast out harmful invaders. Papaya enzymes have been shown to work well in acid, alkaline, and neutral environments.

CORRECTS WRIST AND SHOULDER ARTHRITIS WITH FOOD THERAPY

Retired schoolteacher Sarah R. Y. was concerned when her wrists and shoulders became stiff. She feared arthritis. Her physical therapist outlined a "movement therapy" program which consisted of regular exercise but also urged her to include more garlic and onions in her salads every single day. She was also to use fresh figs and papaya as a dessert. In addition, Sarah R. Y. would follow the aforedescribed nutritional program that worked for Dr. Bingham's thousands of patients. Within six weeks, her stiffness "went away" and she was soon flexible and happy again. Her therapist preferred to believe it was the invigoration of easy exercise plus the garlic-onion-fig-papaya program that prompted the therapeutic immune-building reaction.

You can fight back against arthritis. You can beat the odds against the viral invasion. With the help of nutritional therapy, you can triumph against the so-called "hopeless" condition of arthritis. Feed your immune system and you strengthen your metabolic system to uproot, cast out, and heal your arthritis.

IN REVIEW

1. A leading arthritis specialist physician has found that nutrition will help boost immunity and successfully heal most conditions.
2. Improve your nutritional program with the physician's suggestions as used in his highly acclaimed medical center and rebuild your abused immune system and develop resistance to arthritis.
3. Clifford D. N. speedily overcame his painful arthritis with adjustments in his food program.
4. Four foods may be used daily to nourish your immune system to resist and eradicate arthritis.
5. Sarah R. Y. was healed of wrist and shoulder arthritis with the help of a simple, improved nutritional program and the use of four special and easily available foods.

20

Freedom from Arthritis: Your Lifetime Program

Make life easier for yourself with better self-care while at home, at work, or during routine activities. Do not let arthritis turn you into a bedridden invalid. Too much inactivity prolongs muscle pain. If you continue to rest an injured muscle past the time it needs to heal, the lack of use shortens and stiffens the muscle fibers, worsening the pain when you finally do move.

Muscle fibers start to shorten within a matter of days once you start resting them. Keep your body moving without any strain or pain and you will help oxygenate your immune system to help send forth the important T-cells or lymphocytes to do battle with arthritis invaders.

Here is a set of programs designed to keep your immune system working at full speed while you carry on your daily obligations.

AEROBIC ACTIVITIES ARE REFRESHING

Aerobic exercise is a technical term for any physical activity that improves the conditioning of the heart and lungs by making them work harder than they are used to. Typical aerobic activities include—brisk walking, jogging, swimming, bicycling, cross-country skiing, jumping jacks, jumping rope—whatever it takes to raise your pulse rate and get you to breathe deeply.

Begin and end every aerobic exercise session with a few minutes of stretching and other warmup exercises. Your muscles will be more flexible and less prone to injury during aerobic exercise if you stretch them first. After you've finished exercising, ease your muscles back into a normal routine with a few more minutes of simple exercises.

To be effective, aerobic exercise should be undertaken three or more days each week. Do not plunge in. Start with a few minutes a day and work up to 20 or 30 minutes. The exercise should make you breathe deeply but it should not make you breathless.

FITNESS AT THE WORKSITE

Many folks spend the better part of their waking hours at a workbench or desk. *Problem:* Sitting for hours can be hurtful to your back and lead to muscle strain. *Solution:* Exercise your muscles during the workday.

Take a brisk walk during your lunch hour. Walk up and down stairs instead of taking the elevator. Simply tightening the muscles of your abdomen on and off throughout the day will help tone up those important muscles. Try these movement therapies at the worksite:

*Gently lower your head to relieve blockages in your neck and shoulders. Then raise up and tilt as far back as is comfortable. Repeat several times.

*While seated, bend your upper torso and lower your head between your legs as if searching for something under your seat. Repeat a few times.

*To release tension in your shoulders, upper back, and neck, gently lower your head to stretch and relax the muscles. Hold the position for ten seconds.

*To stretch all the muscles in your back, lean forward in your chair and gently lower your head, shoulders, and arms between your knees. Stay there for ten seconds.

*Stand with your back against a wall and with your heels about 6 inches away from the wall. Flatten your lumbar (lower) curve by pressing the small of your back against the wall and tightening your abdominal muscles. Hold for ten seconds.

*Sit comfortably in your chair and extend one leg out in front of you so that it is parallel with the floor and your foot is perpendicular to the floor. Stretch your entire leg. Then point your toes forward and rotate your foot to make an "O" shape with your toes. Repeat the exercise with the other leg.

STANDING AND WALKING

Standing puts less strain on the back than sitting. You need to do both, of course, so follow the basics of good posture.

*High heels increase the lumbar curve—the higher the heels, the more exaggerated the curve. *Simple Test:* Remove your shoes, stand up and slowly rise up on the balls of your feet. As you do so, concentrate on the muscles in the small of your back. Feel them tightening? As you rise, your legs and the middle of your back are thrust forward. *Tip:* To keep your body from toppling forward, choose shoes that are good for your back as well as your feet.

*Bending forward at the kitchen or bathroom sink can be stressful. When you use the sink, stand comfortably straight with knees slightly flexed. Lean on the sink with one arm for extra support when performing functions that require only one hand, such as brushing your teeth.

*When you must stand a lot in one position, put one foot on a stool or box to reduce the lumbar curve and relieve the stress on your lower back. Alternate feet, and your legs as well, so your back will feel better for it.

*Walk around as much as you can at standup events to keep the strain from building up on your spine.

*Standing and walking with a heavy purse on one shoulder or carrying a heavy briefcase tends to pull the back out of alignment and increase muscle strain. Keep the strain from building up on one side by switching your purse or briefcase back and forth. Better yet, carry a purse or briefcase of more manageable size. When you travel, distribute your baggage between two small or medium-sized suitcases instead of carrying everything in one large, posture-distorting suitcase.

*If you feel tension building in the muscles of your back, try this soothing remedy: lie in a comfortable position on the floor or on your bed, or sit in an upholstered chair that supports your back, head, and arms. If you're lying down, place some pillows under the backs of your knees and another one under your head. Lay your arms at your sides or on the armrests of your chair. Inhale deeply while slowly counting to four; hold your breath for a count of two; exhale slowly while again counting to four. Concentrate only on this slow, deep breathing. Within five to ten minutes, you will feel completely relaxed. Lie or sit there a few more minutes in this stress-free condition before you resume what you were doing.

*When standing, keep your back comfortably straight, your legs slightly flexed, and your buttocks tucked under. If you must stand in one spot for long periods, put one foot on a stool or large book to take the stress off your back.

*Bend your knees when you lift anything from the floor. Hold heavy objects close to you when lifting and carrying them.

*When you carry bundles, distribute the load evenly between two small or medium-sized bags instead of carrying everything in one big posture-hurting bag.

BE GOOD TO YOUR FEET

There are 26 bones and more than 150 ligaments and muscles in your feet and they need special attention. From morning to night, they walk an average of 5 or more miles. With every step, one foot supports twice your body weight. For arthritis-troubled feet, try these simple remedies:

*Alternate between heels and flats to keep tendons flexible. Change shoes and footwear daily to keep your feet dry, healthy, and happy.

*Lie on the floor near a wall. Raise your legs until they're 2 or 3 feet over your head; then rest your feet against the wall. Hold them there for a few minutes; this allows all the blood that's settled in your lower legs and feet to recirculate. For special help, firmly massage your feet and legs upward from ankle to calf.

*Start from a standing position, feet a shoulder's width apart. Pick up the right foot slowly, lifting the heel first, then the ball of the foot, and finally the toes. Meanwhile, shift your weight slowly, until all weight is on your left foot and your right foot is barely off the floor. Repeat five times, then switch feet.

*Sitting in a chair, extend one leg. Point your toes, then flex. Sounds easy but could be done incorrectly. Remember— do *not* curl your toes when you point. The stretch should come in the muscles of the top of the foot, not in the toes.

*Still sitting, rotate your foot slowly at the ankle. Reverse directions. Then do the same for the other foot.

TIPS FOR DRIVERS' FEET

Your feet, ankles, and legs may cramp, swell, or ache from the pressure of keeping them on the pedals of your car during a long trip. Here are simple exercises you can do (try them only when the car is stopped) to help relieve this congestion:

1. Jog by raising your feet alternately as high as possible. This is a warmup to continue for one to three minutes.

2. Extend one leg, point toes, then flex. Repeat five times on each foot.

3. Lift your foot and rotate in circles in each direction 15 times. Repeat on each foot two times. (This exercise is great for swollen ankles.)

4. Massage relaxes tired muscles and boosts immune-feeding circulation. Whether you spend the whole day driving or just some of the day in your car, your feet deserve special attention. Grasp your feet with fingers on top and thumb on sole. Apply firm thumb pressure in a circular motion over the entire sole. Then switch positions, with thumb on top.

BE GOOD TO YOUR KNEES

*Overweight? Shed pounds to help maintain healthy and stress-free knees.

*Avoid excessive squatting or stair-climbing which puts a force seven times your weight across the kneecap. This stress between kneecap and thigh can exceed 2,000 pounds when you stand up. If you must work below your waist, pull up a stool or sit on the floor.

*Gardening? Kneel on a foam cushion and frequently shift your weight. Sit down on the ground periodically to work, but, again, change your leg position often.

*If forced to sit for a long time, keep changing positions. Cross and uncross your legs, slide forward in your seat, stretch your legs, and, whenever possible, get up and walk around.

*If you sit very long, be sure your chair provides proper support for your lower back. Your knees should be slightly higher than your hips and your chair should be big enough for you to shift around in from time to time to alleviate the stress of sitting.

*Minimize strain while driving by adjusting your car seat far enough forward so that you do not have to stretch to reach the wheel and the gas pedal.

*Look for a more resilient surface if you do much walking or other activities. Avoid concrete or wood-over-concrete, which absorb none of the impact which is sent shooting up your legs and knees.

*For fast walking, guard against hyperextending your legs. That is, straightening them to an abnormal degree, because it stretches tendons in the back of your knee and could be hurtful. When walking or running, always keep your knees slightly bent.

EASING ARTHRITIS PAIN WITH HOME REMEDIES

Morning Neck Pain

Sleep on a firm mattress and discard your pillow. For pain, use comfortable heat: via a hot shower, hot compresses, or a heating pad. To improve neck comfort, take a bath towel, fold it lengthwise to about 4 inches of width, and wrap around your neck; fasten with tape or safety pin. Many neck pains are eased by simply supporting your neck. *Careful:* Never turn too quickly or too far.

Shoulder Pain

Congestion is a probable cause with accumulated wastes in the soft tissues near the joint. Try gentle heat or a cold pack. Also, try a pendulum swing. Lean over so your arm hangs like a pendulum and swing around in ever-increasing circles. Try to relax, not tense your neck and upper back muscles when under stress.

Side Stitches

It's a painful catch below your rib cage. Stop whatever you are doing. Breathe it away. Adjust your breathing pattern from deep, rhythmic breathing to shallow, quick breathing or vice versa. *Tip:* Breathing from your diaphragm will build immunity to this minor ache.

Back Pain

A heating pad is comfortable, but try ice. It reduces inflammation and eliminates pain while preventing much of the swelling from occurring. An ice "popsicle" applied to the hurt area for 15 minutes every four to six hours will anesthetize the muscle spasm and ease strain. (To make, freeze a paper cup filled with water and tear off the upper half. Peel remainder as ice melts.)

*If pain and stiffness still remain, especially on awakening, heat is helpful. Watch an old arthritic or rheumatic dog and see how it searches out the sunniest part of the yard to warm its bones. You can learn a new trick from an old dog!

*If you feel an approaching back pain, lie on the floor, your head and buttocks supported by pillows and your legs resting on a chair. Move the trunk of your body as far under the chair as possible. You'll feel much better.

*Do much reading or needlework? Do so with a thick cushion across your lap. It supports the weight of your arms and eases posture pressure; it also eliminates the hurtful chin-on-chest position.

*Arthritic knee pain? Place bags of ice on your knees for 20 minutes, three times a day, to ease pain, give you better movement, and improve joint strength.

*Leg cramps. They sneak up at night and your muscle feels shredded. Do *not* draw up your leg—stretch it. Get up and walk for awhile. Knead or massage like a lump of dough until you feel relaxed. A warm cloth is often calming and softening to a tensed muscle.

*If your feet are stiff but *not* swollen, soak in warm water for 15 minutes once or twice a day. If you have swelling, follow a warm-water soak with two minutes in cool water and repeat. Do this twice a day.

FOUR BASIC PAIN RELIEVERS

1. *Stimulants.* Liniments, hot poultices, massage, and ice packs help stimulate your immune system to set off a response to dilate your blood vessels and provide relief.

2. *Heat.* Whether steam, heat lamp, pack, hot water bottle, etc., it helps relax muscle spasm and relieve pain.

3. *Cold.* Constricts blood vessels to help them dilate.

4. *Bed rest.* Within reason, it reduces the friction and allows muscles to relax. The sleeping surface should allow ease of motion and allow your body, particularly your back, to rest comfortably. Best position? The one that produces the least strain!

* * * *

The modern science of immunology has recognized arthritis as a consequence of an invasion of unwanted viral or bacterial substances. The focus has shifted. There is hope for freedom of arthritis through a rebuilding of the immune system. With the programs outlined in this book, you can expect relief from pain almost from the start. Become dedicated to the programs. Set your sights on your goal—to have a strong immune system and cast out arthritis!

Unlike many arthritics, who do nothing but worry about their condition, you have a variety of nutritional and therapeutic activities that make each day interesting and challenging. You will soon have a positive mental attitude, and youthful energy as you move closer and closer to this goal.

With these programs in your favor, you will help your immune system achieve a healing of arthritis. You can win! You *will* win!!

IN REVIEW

1. Rebuild your body through an exercise-stimulating immune system. It is the cornerstone of freedom from arthritis.

2. Improve your standing, walking, working, driving, and sitting postures. Take the strain off your body.

3. Refer to the home remedies for swift healing of hurt.

4. Build these programs into your daily lifestyle and feel your immune system strengthen to ease and erase arthritis.

5. With the help of an invigorated immune system, you can strike back at arthritis—and win!

GLOSSARY

A

Acetylcholine—A central nervous system neurotransmitter that is released by nerve cells and acts either on other nerve cells or on muscles and organs throughout the body.

Adrenal cortex—A section of the brain that produces most of the chemical substances (i.e., steroids) that regulate your metabolism. It is this section of the brain that is activated by drugs known as adrenocorticoids.

Agammaglobulinemia—Total lack of immunoglobulins.

Allergen—Any substance that causes an allergy.

Allergy—The inappropriate and harmful response of the immune system to normally harmless substances.

Ankylosis—The stiffening of a joint produced by any of several causes ranging from the thickening of fibrous tissue or the wearing away of cartilage.

Ankylosing spondylitis—A type of arthritis that affects the spine; inflammation results in fusing of the bones of the spine, shoulders, hips, and other joints.

Antibody—A protein molecule produced and secreted by certain types of white cells in response to an antigen. Antibodies travel, via the bloodstream, to injured or diseased areas of the body. Their accumulation, along with other body fluids, produces the swelling and redness otherwise known as inflammation.

Antigen—Any substance that provokes an immune response when introduced into the body.

Antioxidant—One of a variety of natural or synthetic substances that can prevent or delay the oxygen-caused deterioration of a molecule. Vegetable oils and many foods and nutrients contain antioxidants.

Atherosclerosis—Narrowing of a blood vessel supplying blood to the brain, usually caused by a buildup of fatty deposits along the inner layers of the vessel walls.

Attenuated—Description of a microbe that has been changed slightly so that it no longer causes disease.

Autoantibody—One that reacts against a person's own tissue.

Autoimmune disease—A condition that results when the body's own immune system produces harmful autoantibodies.

Autoimmune response—An internal reaction in which the body's antibodies attack the body's own cells. This internal "misfiring" is thought to be the underlying cause of rheumatoid arthritis.

B

B-cells—White blood cells of the immune system derived from bone marrow and involved in the production of antibodies; they are also called B-lymphocytes.

Bacterium—Microscopic organism composed of a single cell. Many bacteria can cause disease in humans.

Basophil—A special white blood cell, called a granulocyte, filled with granules of toxic chemicals that can digest microorganisms. Like the mast cell, its counterpart in the tissues, basophils are responsible for hurtful symptoms of arthritis.

Bone marrow—Soft tissue located in the cavities of the bones. Responsible for producing blood cells.

Bursa—The small pouch found in the tissue that connects joints.

Bursitis—Inflammation of the bursa.

C

Calcification—Mineral deposits in muscles and joints that can produce pain, reduce flexibility, and produce an inflammatory response.

Carpal tunnel syndrome—A degenerative inflammation of the wrist.

Cartilage—Tough, dense, gristly material that covers the tip of each bone and protects the end of the bone. The wearing away of the cartilage—thus leaving no protection for the tips of the bones—is the main symptom of osteoarthritis.

Cholesterol—A fat-like substance found in all animal tissues which is believed to contribute to atherosclerosis.

Collagen—A protein substance found in connective tissue throughout the body.

Complement—A complex series of blood proteins involved in the immune response.

Complement cascade—A precise sequence of events, usually triggered by an antigen-antibody complex, in which each component of the complement system is activated in turn, resulting in inflammation and destruction of microbes.

Cortisone—A powerful hormone that in its natural form is produced by the adrenal glands. It works by producing significant changes in the metabolism.

D

DNA—Deoxyribonucleic acid is the genetic material of all cells. Composed of a chain of nitrogen-based subunits (nucleic acids) found in the chromosomes of a cell.

Docosahexaenoic acid (DHA)—An Omega-3 fatty acid found in fish, fish oils, and the fat of marine mammals who live on fish; believed to have immune-boosting properties.

E

Eicosapentaenoic acid (EPA)—An Omega-3 fatty acid, same as DHA.

Endorphin—A group of chemical substances. The body's own opiate neuropeptides produced by the brain. Has a morphine-like action. The chain of amino acids acts on the nervous system to reduce pain. The body's own weapon to relieve pain.

Enkephalin—Like endorphin, a naturally produced chemical that has a soothing or morphine-like action. Usually found in the brain and spinal cord; its action is analogous to that of the endorphins.

Eosinophil—A special white blood cell, called a granulocyte, that can digest harmful microorganisms. Plays a role in arthritis reactions.

Epitope—A characteristic shape or marker on an antigen's surface.

F

Fibrositis—A condition in which there is generalized pain in the muscles, ligaments, and tendons.

G

Gout—A systemic, metabolic condition that produces swelling and pain in the big toe and other joints in the foot. It occurs when the body is unable to properly use uric acid. An excess forms needle-like crystals in the joints and leads to severe inflammation.

Granulocytes—A cell of the immune system filled with granules of toxic chemicals that enable them to digest microorganisms. Basophils, neutrophils, eosinophils, and mast cells are examples of granulocytes.

H

Heberden's nodes—Bony growths in the finger joints closest to the nails; associated with osteoarthritis.

Helper T-cells—A subset of T-cells that turn on antibody production.

Hypogammaglobulinemia—Lower than normal levels of immuno-globulins.

I

Immune complex—Large molecules formed when antigen and anti-body bind together.
Immune response—The activity of the immune system against foreign substances or antigens.
Immunocompetent—Capacity to develop an immune response.
Immunogen—A term used to describe any substance that elicits an immune response.
Immunoglobulin—Another name for antibody.
Infectious arthritis—A form of arthritis whose underlying causes are bacteria, viruses, or fungi. It can affect any joint.
Inflammation—A reaction of the body to injury or disease, causing pain, swelling, redness, warmth, and sometimes loss of motion in the area affected.

J

Joint—Any place in the body where two bones come together.

L

Leukocytes—The white blood cells.
Ligament—A strong, cord-like elastic structure that connects bones to other bones and holds the joint in place.
Lipid peroxidation—The process in which oxygen-free radicals attack the fatty outer coating (membrane) of the cells. Lipid peroxides formed from normal lipids (fats) of the cell membrane or body are unable to perform the necessary metabolic and structural roles that fats ordinarily play.
Lipofuscins—A class of fatty pigments consisting mostly of oxidized fats that are found in abundance in the cells of adults. Some studies suggest that lipofuscins are responsible for the aging process in a cell.
Lymph—A transparent, slightly yellow fluid containing primarily lymphocytes. Lymph is composed of tissue fluids collected from all parts of the body and returned to the blood via the lymphatic vessels.
Lymph nodes—Small, bean-sized organs of the immune system, distributed widely throughout the body. An outpost for B-lympho-cytes.

Lymphocytes—Small white cells, normally present in the blood and in lymphoid tissue, that bear the major responsibility of carrying out the functions of the immune system.

Lymphokines—Powerful substances produced and released into the bloodstream by T-lymphocytes and capable of stimulating other cells in the immune system.

M

Macrophage—A scavenger cell found in the tissues; able to destroy invading bacteria or other foreign material. Larger than normal white cells that are part of the immune system. They operate by, in effect, "swallowing" bacteria, antigens, and viruses.

Mast cells—Special cells found in the tissues; contain granules of chemicals responsible for the symptoms of arthritis outbreak.

Microbes—Minute living organisms, including bacteria, protozoa, and fungi.

Microorganism—Any microscopic plant or animal.

Molecule—The smallest unit of matter of an element or compound.

Monocyte—A large white blood cell that acts as a scavenger, capable of destroying invading bacteria or other foreign material.

Monokines—Powerful chemical substances that are secreted by macrophages and monocytes and help direct and regulate the immune response.

N

Natural killer cells—Large granular lymphocytes that attack and destroy other cells such as arthritic cells and those infected with viruses or other microbes.

Neuron—The basic nerve cells of the nervous system containing a nucleus within a cell body; an axon (trunk-like projection containing neurotransmitter molecules) and dendrites (branched projections containing receptor sites.)

Neurotransmitters—Molecules that carry chemical messages between nerve cells. Neurotransmitters are released from a neuron, diffuse across the minute space between cells (synaptic cleft), and bind to a receptor located on the post-synaptic neuron.

Neutrophil—Granular white blood cell, called a granulocyte, that participates in the immune response to a foreign substance and can digest harmful microorganisms. Part of the body's defense system to produce oxygen radicals to destroy invaders.

O

Omega-3 fatty acid—A fatty acid chain which has its first double bond starting on the third carbon atom of the chain.

Osteoarthritis—The most common form of arthritis; generally results from wear and tear in the mechanical parts of the joint. Commonly affects weight-bearing joints such as hips, knees, and ankles.

Osteoporosis—A medical disorder characterized by the softening of the bones, due to the loss of calcium. Although not strictly a form of arthritis, it is nonetheless associated with many types of arthritis.

Oxidation—Refers to the state of being oxidized or the act of oxidizing another substance. A molecule is oxidized when it loses electrons (negative charges); thus it becomes more positively charged. Oxidation is always coupled with reduction (gain of electrons)—one atom loses electrons, another gains them.

Oxygen-free radicals—Highly reactive (due to an unpaired electron) and unstable byproducts of oxygen metabolism with extremely short half-lives and capable of causing damage or death to cells.

P

Periostitis—An inflammation of the membrane surrounding the bone.

Plasma cells—Antibody-producing cells descended from B-cells.

Phagocytes—A category of protective white cells that can ingest and digest microorganisms or other foreign substances. They ingest body debris; phagocytes release oxygen radicals when they engulf foreign matter.

Physiatrist—A medical doctor specializing in physical medicine and rehabilitation.

Placebo—An inactive substance the person takes, believing it has medical properties.

Polyarthritis—Inflammation affecting several joints at the same time.

Prostaglandins—A category of chemical substances found throughout the body and believed to play a central role in the two principal symptoms of arthritis: pain and inflammation. Prostaglandins accelerate the movement of antibodies to diseased or injured areas and trigger the nerve action that underlies pain. It is through the inhibition of prostaglandin production that aspirin and non-steroid anti-inflammatory drugs are able to control pain and inflammation.

R

Reynaud's phenomenon—An internal reaction triggered by either climate or an emotional response; it temporarily cuts off the blood flow to the extremities, resulting in numbness and pain.

Rheumatoid arthritis—While it can affect the entire body, the joints most commonly involved are those of the hands and feet; believed caused by a defect of the body's own defense or immune system. Has an inflammatory nature.

RNA—Ribonucleic acid, found in all living cells; transmits information from DNA to the protein-forming system of the cell. RNA is composed of a chain of nitrogen-based subunits (nucleic acids).

S

Salicylates—A family of chemicals capable of reducing pain, fever, and inflammation. Aspirin is a common member.

Scavenger—A substance that can combine with an absorbing electron from free radicals, thereby protecting cells or other invaders from hurtful attack.

Scavenger cells—Any of a diverse group of cells that have the capacity to engulf and destroy foreign material, dead cells, or tissues.

Scleroderma—A rheumatic disease whose chief symptom is a hardening of collagen, the connective tissue surrounding most joints. This thickening and hardening along with inflammation can occur in internal organs, the esophagus, intestinal tract, heart, lungs, and kidneys.

Sedimentation—Also known as the sed rate. This term refers to the settling of red blood cells by gravity. The rate of settling is an index of circulating inflammatory proteins.

Serotonin—A neurotransmitter thought to play a role in temperature regulation, mood, and sleep. Found in the brain as well as in the circulating blood.

Spleen—An organ in the abdominal cavity; an important source of antibody production.

Stern cells—Cells from which all blood cells derive energy.

Steroids—Hormones produced by the adrenal cortex. Their prime functions are to regulate metabolism, maintain blood pressure, and control sexual appearance and behavior.

Superoxide—A common and reactive form of oxygen ($O2''$) in biological reactions that is formed when molecular oxygen gains a single electron. Superoxide radicals can attack susceptible biological targets (lipids, proteins, nucleic acids).

Superoxide dismutase (SOD)—An enzyme found in many cells that converts superoxide radicals to less toxic agents.

Suppressor T-cells—Subset of T-cells that "turn off" antibody production.

Synapse—The minute space between two neurons or between a neuron and an organ across which nerve impulses are chemically transmitted.

Synovial membrane—The thin membrane that lines most of the joints in the body, particularly those in the hands, feet, wrists, elbows, and shoulders. Its function is to protect the joint and to secrete synovial fluid that "oils" the joint. The thickening and inflammation of synovial tissue is the principal symptom of rheumatoid arthritis.

Systemic disease—One that can affect many parts of the body, not only a small area.

Systemic lupus erythematosus or SLE—Also known as "lupus," a rheumatic disease that involves, inflames, and damages body tissues; these include the skin, joints, and internal organs. SLE is believed caused when something triggers the immune system to turn against the body.

T

T-cells—White blood cells produced by the thymus; they further produce lymphokines and play an important part in the body's ability to fight viruses and bacteria. Also called T-lymphocytes.

Tendinitis—Inflammation of a tendon.

Tendon—The strong, cord-like, tapered end of a muscle that connects the muscle to a bone.

Thymus—A central lymphoid organ important in the development of immune capability.

Triglycerides—Glyceride particles formed during the process of digesting dietary fats. High levels of serum triglycerides have been shown to be responsible for a clogging of the immune system.

V

Vaccine—A substance that contains the antigen of an organism and stimulates active immunity; provides future protection against infection by that organism.

Virus—Submicroscopic microbe causing infectious disease. Can reproduce only in living cells.

Index

269